CIRCUIT RIDERS FOR MENTAL HEALTH

CIRCUIT RIDERS *for* MENTAL HEALTH

The Hogg Foundation in Twentieth-Century Texas

WILLIAM S. BUSH

Texas A&M University Press
College Station

First edition

This paper meets the requirements of ANSI/NISO Z39.48-1992 (Permanence of Paper).
Binding materials have been chosen for durability.

Manufactured in the United States of America

Library of Congress Cataloging-in-Publication Data

Names: Bush, William S., 1967–, author
Title: Circuit riders for mental health: the Hogg Foundation in twentieth-century Texas / William S. Bush.
Description: First edition. | College Station: Texas A&M University Press, 2016. | Includes bibliographical references and index.
Identifiers: LCCN 2016009097 (print) | LCCN 2016012334 (ebook) | ISBN 9781623494445 (cloth: alk. paper) | ISBN 9781623494452 (ebook)
Subjects: LCSH: Hogg Foundation for Mental Health—History—20th century. | Mental health services—Texas—History—20th century. | Mental health policy—Texas—History—20th century. | Mentally ill—Care—Texas—History—20th century.
Classification: LCC RA790.65.T4 B87 2016 (print) | LCC RA790.65.T4 (ebook) | DDC 362.209764—dc23

LC record available at http://lccn.loc.gov/2016009097

For Mary, Alex, and Ollie

Contents

Illustrations

Acknowledgments

This book began as a vague idea over a decade ago during conversations with King Davis, a member of my dissertation committee at the University of Texas and at that time the executive director of the Hogg Foundation. He persuaded me that an untold story of mental health reform called for historical attention. Other projects beckoned, however, and I put this one aside at that time.

Years later, I returned to this project with the support of a grant from the Hogg Foundation. I owe a tremendous debt to the Foundation, its leadership, and its staff for their constant support and, importantly, their respect for my freedom to follow the source materials wherever they led. In particular, Octavio Martinez, Lynda Frost, and Dan Oppenheimer have given unflagging support throughout the conception, research, and writing of this book. Lynda Frost's feedback on early chapter drafts proved invaluable. I cannot express my gratitude strongly enough to the ex-staff members who generously shared their personal and professional memories with me during lengthy oral interviews: Wayne Holtzman, Louise and the late Ira Iscoe, Ralph Culler, Reymundo Rodríguez, Robert Leon, Adrian Fowler, and King Davis. I am also grateful for the generosity of Lucille DiDomenico of Philanthropy Southwest (formerly the Conference of Southwest Foundations), who shared documents and photographs in addition to her reminiscences.

My deepest gratitude goes to Victoria Hill, my former colleague in the Department of American Studies at the University of Texas, who served as a research assistant on this project. Vicky and I collaborated closely on the archival research for this project and held numerous extended discussions about the larger questions raised by our source materials. She offered indispensable insights into the history of psychology, the politics of mental health, and the ways in which race and gender surfaced throughout the drama of mental health reform in Texas. Because this book draws heavily on archival records, it has depended crucially on the assistance of archivists and library professionals. In particular I wish to thank Laura Saegert at the Texas State Library and Archives and all of the staff at the Dolph Briscoe Center for American History at the University of Texas at Austin. The librarians on my own campus at Texas A&M University–San Antonio, led by the inimitable Stefanie Wittenbach, provided excellent support. At Texas A&M University Press, my editor Jay Dew has provided expert guidance throughout the manuscript review and production process, and I wish to thank the blind reviewers for their thoughtful feedback on the manuscript.

I also owe thanks to numerous scholarly colleagues, starting with my exceptional colleagues in the History Department at Texas A&M University–San Antonio. Amy Porter, Ed Westermann, and Francis Galan, with whom it is an honor to work, provided helpful commentary on portions of this book manuscript. One of my former mentors at the University of Texas at Austin, Janet Davis, shared some helpful guidance during a critical juncture in this project, for which I am very grateful. Another former colleague, Claytee White, who directs the Oral History Research Center at the University of Nevada–Las Vegas, advised me on key nuances in planning and executing oral interviews. Conversations with mental health professionals helped me understand the changing terminologies and practices that have emerged in recent years. In particular, I wish to thank the aforementioned Lynda Frost as well as Chris Laguna for their insights.

From its earliest years, the mental health movement has highlighted the importance of healthy, nurturing family relationships. I am incredibly blessed to have such a family with my wife, Mary Wright, and our two sons, Alexander and Oliver. Their unfailing love and patience propelled me throughout the completion of this book and inspires me every day.

CIRCUIT RIDERS FOR MENTAL HEALTH

INTRODUCTION

Out of Sight, Out of Mind

One evening in January 2015, a seventeen-year-old woman named Kristiana Coignard walked into a police station in Longview, Texas, and requested to speak with a police officer. When three officers arrived in the lobby, they noticed that Coignard had a kitchen knife in her belt and the words "I Have a Gun" written on her hand. Video surveillance subsequently released to the public showed a sequence of events that lasted for about twenty minutes. In the video, Coignard can be seen being restrained and then released, brandishing her knife at the officers, and finally charging the officers with the knife in hand. The incident ended with multiple gunshots to Coignard's chest, resulting in her death. Media reports expressed confusion over the reasons for Coignard's actions and outrage at what many perceived as an excessive use of force. Coignard's lack of a criminal record or any history of violent behavior caused some observers to lump the incident in with other controversial police shootings of civilians in Ferguson, Missouri, and New York City. As it had in those more notorious cases, the hacker group Anonymous launched a cyber-attack against the Longview police department's website; in fact, several of the Longview city agency websites were hacked and unavailable as a result. The release of video footage of the incident did little to quell matters. Indeed, after viewing the Longview police video, Coignard's father, a former correctional officer himself, lambasted the officers for their inability to restrain his teenage daughter without the use of firearms. The officers "shouldn't have allowed the situation to escalate the way it did," he concluded. "My daughter should still be alive."[1]

Within days of the shooting, it was reported that Coignard had lived with mental illness for much of her brief life. In an interview given to the website Think Progress, Coignard's aunt revealed that her biological mother had died when she was four years old and that she had struggled with bipolar disorder and depression for "most of her life." A native of San Antonio, Coignard had been hospitalized twice following suicide attempts and had moved to her grandparents' home in Longview only a few months before her death. According to her relatives, Coignard had appeared to improve after the move. She had begun seeing a therapist, who had prescribed behavioral medication, had earned her general education diploma, and had taken a job at a local restaurant. Nevertheless, something had prompted Coignard to walk into the Longview police station that fateful evening. Her aunt characterized the incident as "a cry for help" that need not have ended so tragically, recounting that, until that evening, Coignard "was only violent with herself."[2] Months after Coignard's death, the police released a handwritten suicide note found in her backpack that read, in part,

> This is no one's fault but my own. I've tried getting help, but it never worked. Things would seem to get better, just to get twice as bad. My mental health is a joke; I don't deserve to live. . . . I'm mentally ill and by removing myself from society, I am doing everyone a favor. This is the right choice. I can't take it anymore.[3]

Critics were quick to point out that the police need not have obliged Coignard's apparent intent. One writer suggested that Coignard's death was not only tragic but "tragically unexceptional," one of "more than a dozen" encounters between police and civilians with mental illness in the previous year that ended with the civilian being fatally shot.[4] While praising the growing use of mental health training in police departments, a spokesperson for the National Alliance on Mental Illness lamented the lack of adequate mental health services in local communities, which, in her view, fueled tragic encounters like the one in Longview. According to the National Institute of Mental Health, Coignard was one of more than 6 million Americans diagnosed with bipolar disorder, and one-quarter of all Americans (61 million) had experienced an episode of mental illness during the previous year. Moreover, Coignard's ability to see a therapist made her exceptional; more than 60 percent of all adults with mental illness had received no mental health services at all during the previous year.[5]

Individuals with mental illness, such as Kristiana Coignard, often live out of sight unless a terrible circumstance brings them into the public consciousness. A little over two years earlier, a series of tragic incidents, punctuated by the mass shooting at Sandy Hook Elementary School in Newtown, Connecticut, sounded a clarion call for greater attention to mental health services. Around the nation, state legislatures sprang into action, voting for dramatic increases in funding for mental health. In Coignard's home state of Texas, the legislature during its 2013 session approved an unprecedented increase of $300 million for mental health services, which represented a 15 percent expansion of the overall budget. Although praised by advocacy groups, this measure generally restored funds that had been cut in previous sessions. Prior to the increase, Texas had ranked "dead last" nationally in per-capita spending on mental health services, and even now it remains well below the national average.[6]

Equally as concerning for mental health advocates has been the Texas Mental Health Code, a set of legal guidelines protecting the civil rights of people with mental illness and setting forth rules and best practices for their treatment. First enacted in 1957, the mental health code had not been substantially updated since 1985. In the meantime, the state's organizational structures, professional terminologies, and standard practices had changed substantially. The lack of appropriate guidelines, combined with inadequate resources, has prevented many individuals from accessing mental health services and caused some to end up in the criminal justice system as a result. In September 2012, the nonprofit groups Texas Appleseed and Disability Rights Texas published a report recommending a complete overhaul of the mental health code.[7] Authored by legal and mental health experts, the report led to legislation expanding the list of diagnostic categories that could qualify for mental health services, among other reforms. One observer called it "possibly the most significant change to the [mental health] system in over a quarter century."[8]

This report was historic not only for its content but also for the process by which it was developed. It was supported by a two-year grant from the Hogg Foundation for Mental Health, an organization founded in 1940 with a mission to "improve the mental health of all Texans." This mission had propelled the Foundation into a decades-long campaign to reform the system of mental health services in Texas and in the process to educate the general public about mental health and mental illness. One of the Foundation's time-honored methods was to send experts around the state, "circuit riders" as they called themselves, educating ordinary people, professionals, and paraprofessionals about mental health, while also listening to their concerns about their lives, their loved ones, and the services and policies they believed would allow them to lead productive lives with dignity and self-respect. Similarly, the 2012 report's authors had conducted more than forty open forums around the state soliciting suggestions for changes to the mental health code. They heard from "consumers, family members, mental health professionals and administrators, hospital administrators, lawyers, advocates, and many others."[9] These groups raised issues broadly resembling those that had animated earlier generations of mental health reformers: unclear requirements for voluntary and involuntary admission to mental health facilities, outdated terminology particularly for diagnostic categories of mental illness, and overuse of the criminal justice system to house individuals with mental illness.

The human toll of these ongoing problems raises important historical questions that this book seeks to answer, starting with the most obvious: Has it always been this way? Contemporary discourses surrounding mental health and mental illness typically express impatience with slow progress toward more robust services, humane policies, and ultimately better outcomes. As one journalist lamented recently, "Texas' system of caring for people with mental illness has never been stellar."[10] Such statements reflect long-standing historical concerns of mental health reformers that this book traces back across the previous century. At the same time, the recent critiques from mental health advocates imply a static and therefore somewhat misleading history. Mental health services in Texas and the nation have changed dramatically since they first emerged nearly two hundred years ago and can lend important context to contemporary discussions. Indeed, what constitutes a "better outcome" today differs markedly from fifty years or two centuries ago. Today, the Texas Department of State Health Service's Substance Abuse and Mental Health Services Administration defines "recovery" as "a process of change through which individuals improve their health and wellness, live a self-directed life, and strive to reach their full potential."[11] Where experts in earlier periods (including those at the Hogg Foundation) might have promoted the notion of "curing" mental illness wholesale, today's proponents speak of "living with mental illness," preferably within their home communities wherever possible. Indeed, the very language used to describe mental health and mental illness has transformed over time. Nineteenth-century psychiatrists named individuals with mental illness as "insane," "mad," or "incurably insane." For much of the twentieth century, one spoke of "the mentally ill" or described individuals with specific conditions as, for instance, "schizophrenic." In recent years, mental health advocates and practitioners speak of people with mental illness as "survivors" or as "consumers" of mental health services. These terms aim to promote respect for individuals' lived experiences, but they also intentionally imply agency. Far more than passive recipients of mental health services, "consumers" are envisioned as active participants in the development of individual treatment plans as well as broader service programming and even public policy.[12]

This transformation is remarkable when considered against the broader history of mental health and mental illness. The organized treatment of mental illness in the United States began in the early nineteenth century, a period when many states opened asylums to house individuals who at the time were understood to be suffering from insanity. In the years prior to the Civil War, the asylum constituted a response to rapid population growth and urbanization, which rendered obsolete informal practices of caring for individuals with mental illness. In addition, the asylum reflected the growing influence of a mode of scientific inquiry that traced its roots to the Enlightenment, as well as a cultural shift propelled by the Second Great Awakening, in which new faith traditions began to reject old-line Protestant notions of individual human depravity in favor of a more optimistic belief in self-improvement.[13] As the historian David J. Rothman has shown in his foundational study, *The Discovery of the Asylum*, psychiatrists in antebellum America believed the asylum offered a controlled environment for the development of "cures" for various forms of mental illness, which at that time was understood as a type of disease requiring expert medical treatment. Led by Dorothea Dix, proponents of the asylum "confidently and aggressively asserted that properly organized institutions could cure almost every instance of the disease."[14] By the 1870s, according to Rothman, the reformers' vision had collapsed; their notion that order and discipline could cure the "recently insane" proved inaccurate. Not only were asylums receiving more chronically and seriously ill patients, even individuals with less serious forms of mental illness did not respond as reformers had hoped.[15] As a result, asylums devolved into largely custodial institutions, a situation that persisted into the early twentieth century, even as many state asylums changed their names to "hospitals" to underscore further their ostensible role as curative rather than custodial institutions. Even state-of-the-art facilities such as Northampton State Hospital in Massachusetts fell into this mold, offering modes of "therapy" that had no proven effectiveness in improving mental illness. These measures included hydrotherapy (e.g., hot baths), the use of restraints, occupational therapies that largely consisted of institution-maintaining labor, and arts and crafts activities; some institutions experimented with drug therapies but to little avail. By the time of World War II, the American mental hospital had acquired a grim reputation that extended to the public's understanding of individuals with mental illness and indeed of mental illness itself.[16]

A similar historical path was followed in Texas, which, like many other Southern states, began opening asylums just before or during the Civil War. Opened in 1861, the Texas State Lunatic Asylum was physically and programmatically modeled closely on the principles of the national movement for asylums. Renamed the Austin State Hospital in 1925, the institution suffered from overcrowding and underfunding throughout most of its existence. Like other American asylums, its original mission of "curing" mental illness quickly gave way to the creation of "a complex society" of patients, administrators, and staff members, countless hundreds of whom lived out their lives inside the institution's walls over the institution's first century of existence.[17] This story is chronicled in *Life at the Texas State Lunatic Asylum, 1857–1997*, which remains to date the only published history of mental health and mental illness in Texas.

Amid the renaming of asylums as mental hospitals in the early twentieth century, a new reform movement emerged that questioned the bedrock assumptions behind large institutions for people with mental illness. Led by psychiatrists, psychologists, social workers, and former hospital patients ("survivors" in contemporary language), this movement denounced mental hospitals as ineffective and abusive and insisted that the majority of patients could and should reside in their home communities. To do so would require new community-based services and a wholesale transformation in social conceptions of mental illness. The very name of the movement—"mental hygiene"—sought to drive home these points. Its proponents argued that mental health and mental illness existed on a continuum shared by all individuals, and therefore the fostering of mental hygiene or "positive mental health" formed a wider imperative for society. This movement propelled a host of national transformations in mental health policies and services across the twentieth century. In the vanguard of this movement in Texas was the Hogg Foundation for Mental Health, an organization that for nearly three decades acted as the driving force behind sweeping changes in popular understandings of mental health and mental illness, public policy reforms in the provision of institutional and community-based services, the professionalization of mental health services, and the expansion of access to mental health services to historically neglected populations. When the Hogg Foundation began work in 1940, it confronted a scene dominated by dilapidated, prison-like mental hospitals scattered around the state. These institutions provided nearly all the mental health services in the state, outside of a small number of child guidance clinics founded in the interwar era and a few private practitioners of psychiatry. Academic and professional programs in related disciplines were few and far between, while the average Texan associated "mental health" with "insanity" and the "loony bin," as one Hogg Foundation consultant observed in the 1950s (described in chapter 5).

This book chronicles the transformation of this bleak landscape into a vibrant terrain where advocates now more fully include individuals with mental illness and where custody is widely understood to pale in importance to autonomy, dignity, and self-respect. It focuses on the history of mental health rather than mental illness and thus examines a broad range of actors in addition to the psychiatrists and psychologists who often take center stage in histories of mental illness. The story unfolds across six chapters, each of which is told through the lens of the Hogg Foundation, which formed the lead actor in the drama of mental health reform in Texas from 1940 into the mid-1970s. Chapter 1 begins with the Hogg family's early interest in mental health and mental illness during the governorship of James Stephen Hogg in the 1890s, focusing particularly on his only daughter, Ima Hogg, who was herself a "consumer" of mental health services in the 1910s and 1920s. Ima experienced serious depression and visited with several experts, who introduced her to the national mental hygiene movement and made her into a strong believer in the need for widely available mental health services. The chapter describes Ima's attempts to initiate those services in Texas, culminating with the founding of the Hogg Foundation for Mental Hygiene in 1940. The Foundation was unique for its time: a private philanthropy administered through a public university, the University of Texas at Austin, and the first foundation in the nation devoted exclusively to mental health. The Foundation's first order of business was educating the public on mental health. Chapter 2 portrays the excursions of a cohort of "circuit riders" into Texas' cities, small towns, and unincorporated areas to deliver the message of mental health before various audiences in the 1940s and early 1950s. These visits thrust Foundation spokespersons into the middle of thorny social and cultural controversies surrounding gender roles, sexual mores, and race relations and thus shed new light on the ways in which mental health reform helped modernize everyday life in twentieth-century Texas.

Leading the way was the Foundation's inaugural director, Robert Lee Sutherland, an influential yet enigmatic figure who astutely parlayed the Foundation's relatively modest endowment into an influential force through a combination of massive public outreach and smartly forged political and professional alliances. The former is described in chapter 2, while the latter forms the bulk of the discussion in chapter 3, which uncovers the Foundation's key but untold role in the enactment of sweeping reforms of the state's mental hospitals, the provision of state-supported community mental health services, and the establishment of the first Texas Mental Health Code in the 1950s. The lengthy campaign began behind the scenes almost immediately after Sutherland's arrival in Texas in 1940 and burst into the news headlines a decade later, amid a national outcry against custodial institutions for people with mental illness. Widely viewed as constituting a "revolution" in mental health, the reforms of the 1950s reflected an expanding field for mental health philanthropy and research, which form the subject of chapter 4. A sudden and substantial increase in the Foundation's endowment fueled the emergence of a regional network of foundations, the Conference of Southwest Foundations, which allowed for even greater support of mental health reforms. The Foundation also began supporting a research monograph series that expanded the field of mental health services into such areas as disaster relief, psychological testing, and cross-cultural psychology. The entrance of mental health into the mainstream of American life drew a backlash from anticommunists, who attacked the Foundation specifically and mental health generally as a communist "brainwashing" conspiracy, which had a long-term chilling effect on the Foundation's public policy activity.

That effect would not appear immediately, however, as chapter 5 illustrates in its discussion of the full emergence of community mental health services in the 1960s. The Foundation played a key role in the writing of the Texas Plan for Mental Health, supported by federal legislation and which followed up on the Foundation-led reforms of the previous decade mandating more community rather than institutional services for people with mental illness. The Texas Plan formed the basis for the creation of the Texas Department of Mental Health and Mental Retardation, the first statewide agency of its kind in Texas history and a watershed moment for community mental health. Closer to home, the Foundation led in the response to the notorious mass shooting that took place at the University of Texas in August 1966. Informed by the principles of community mental health, the Foundation developed one of the most extensive student counseling services in the state and nation, forecasting some of the priorities that have become normative in the mental health field today. With these achievements, the Foundation found itself in a new world by the end of the 1960s, no longer the only or even the largest actor in the state's mental health scene. Chapter 6 provides a coda to this critical period in the history of mental health and of the Hogg Foundation by examining a new wave of "circuit riding," this time into minority communities led by the Rio Grande Valley in the 1970s. It concludes by exploring the Foundation's shifting priorities in the 1980s and 1990s amid a more complex landscape of mental health services and policies.

On the occasion of the Hogg Foundation's seventy-fifth anniversary, it is noteworthy that one of the public's first responses to tragic incidents such as that of Kristiana Coignard is to inquire into the possibility of mental illness. A public dialogue that is largely empathetic and compassionate represents a testimonial to the success of over a half-century of public education, advocacy, and social change. On the other hand, the continued lament over inadequate services in the community, and seeming public apathy to the legislation and resource needs to provide those services, suggests something quite different. Amid these cross-currents, it seems an opportune moment to revisit this history, if for no other reason than to remind ourselves that mental health has never truly been out of our collective sight or mind.

1

"A Mental Health Program for the People of Texas"

The Birth of the Hogg Foundation

On the evening of Wednesday, February 12, 1941, the president of the University of Texas, Homer Price Rainey, took the stage of the university's Hogg Auditorium. He was there to moderate the formal inauguration ceremony of the Hogg Foundation for Mental Hygiene. In the audience were university faculty, elected and appointed state officials, members of the news media, prominent Texas philanthropists, and nationally recognized experts in the emerging field of mental health. Rainey told his audience that they were present for "some real history in the making" that night. The new Hogg Foundation, he explained, "is going to play the most important role in the redirection of education for the next 20 years—mental health for the normal man."[1] Rainey was hardly alone in holding this seemingly grandiose view. Public anticipation of the Foundation's inauguration had been building for nearly two years, ever since the announcement in July 1939 that the Hogg family had made a $2.5 million bequest to establish a "mental health program" at the state's flagship university. "I am one of thousands who feel an overwhelming gratitude to the Hogg family," read one of the many letters that arrived to Ima Hogg during the summer of 1939.[2] "I was really stunned with joy upon reading the announcement in connection with the Hogg Foundation," wrote Leopold Meyer, a Houston philanthropist and businessman who had collaborated with Ima on other charitable enterprises.[3] Prominent Texas expatriates, led by Minnie Fisher Cunningham of the General Federation of Women's Clubs, sent their congratulations on the establishment of the foundation. Meanwhile, H.T. Manuel, president of the Texas Society for Mental Hygiene, touted the bequest as "the most significant event in Texas during the past year."[4] During the year prior to the inaugural ceremony, President Rainey fielded a steady stream of inquiries from all over Texas, as well as some from other parts of the country. The writers were graduate students, university professors, doctors, psychiatrists, social workers, members of community groups in Texas, researchers in Chicago, professionals in Los

Angeles and Boston, and private citizens from across Texas. Some of the writers sought jobs; others requested in-service training, expressed their desire to enroll in university courses on mental health, requested educational literature on mental health, or eagerly requested more information about the new foundation.[5] Faculty members from universities in and outside of Texas sent their curricula vitae.[6] William H. Jones, dean at all-black Tillotson College in Austin, wrote to recommend Mortelia Womack, a graduate of Fisk University, who was "the only Negro social worker in the Texas State Hospital here in Austin."[7] A member of the El Paso Board of Education wrote requesting assistance from the new foundation for a recently launched child guidance clinic, while a sociology professor from Mary Hardin Baylor College recommended one of his recent graduates for employment (even though no job openings had been listed for the as yet unformed foundation).[8] Clearly, the coming of the Foundation had tapped into a wellspring of excitement, as expressed in one handwritten letter:

> I almost can't believe this wonderful news. I am only twenty-three years old, a recent college graduate—but I *know* the need and value of such a program. I just thrill to think that Texas will enjoy the privileges of this work. I want to have a part in it. I want to work—and I have long yearned, really, to be allowed to enter this type of work. I know that I haven't the necessary specialized training and experience for the technical, scientific side of the work, but isn't there *something* I could do?[9]

The ceremony thus held different meanings for its varied participants. For its hosts at the University of Texas, it announced a new financial endowment from a prominent Texas family. Other observers looked to the new foundation as a source of support for social reform, not only for its stated purpose to promote "mental hygiene for the people of Texas" but for its association with the Hogg family. In the decades immediately preceding the Foundation's establishment, the Hogg family had built a reputation for deploying its wealth for the public good. The principal donor for the Foundation, Will C. Hogg, was a noted philanthropist and one of the university's most prominent alumni. As a privately endowed philanthropy housed within a public university, the Foundation was structurally unique; it also stood out as the only organization of its kind at the time to be devoted solely to mental health. The university affiliation allowed the Foundation to leverage the expertise, reputation, and resources of the university to make the most of its initially modest operating budget. The Foundation embodied a particular philosophy often expressed by the Hogg family generally, and one of its members in particular, whose personal history shaped the decision to devote a portion of the family's fortune to mental health.

The Hogg Family and Mental Health

The driving force behind the Hogg Foundation was Ima Hogg, known to nearly everyone around her as "Miss Ima." Born on July 10, 1882, as the second of four children (Will, born 1875; Mike, born 1885; and Tom, born 1887), and the only daughter, of James Stephen and Sallie Stinson Hogg, Ima grew up within a family committed to "duty to family and responsibility to community."[10] Ima's parents named her in honor of James's oldest brother, Thomas Elisha Hogg, a Civil War veteran and poet. "Ima" was a heroine in "The Fate of Marvin," Thomas's epic poem about the war. Her birthplace, Mineola, was a railroad town where her father James, then an attorney for the Seventh District of Texas, had gained a reputation as a crusading litigator against railroad corporations and banks—"the interests"—all while building a political career in the state Democratic Party. While James Hogg inhabited the rough-and-tumble world of public life, Ima's mother Sallie Stinson Hogg, by all accounts, served the traditional nineteenth-century role as the "civilizing force" in the home, imbuing her children with good morals and good taste in everything from home furnishings to manners. Physically and temperamentally, the couple appeared to be a study in contrasts: the six-foot-three, two- to three-hundred-pound James, with his booming voice and outgoing personality and colorful family history dating back to the era of the Texas Republic, and Sallie, the "five-foot-two, petite," soft-spoken, proper Victorian daughter of a sawmill owner from Quitman, Texas. However, the most recent study of the Hogg family has suggested that these contrasts are misleading. Idealized Victorian portrayals of Sallie, many of them put forth by Ima, have overlooked her "steely determination," her partnership with husband James in managing family and business affairs, and her willingness to balance traditionally strict parenting with more emotional and indulgent childrearing. Many questions remain about James and Sallie, in part due to Ima herself, who kept most of the family records and protected her family's legacy from historical criticism. One thing that is clear, however, is that Ima, as well as her older brother Will, imbibed deeply of her parents' commitment to public service: James, in his various public offices and the positions he took on social issues of the day, and Sallie, in her teachings in the home, which were inspired by the social gospel prevalent at the time. She taught the Hogg children that "they must nurture the communities that had nurtured them."[11]

In 1886 the Hogg family moved to Austin, where Ima would come of age at the center of Texas political life. Her father would go on to serve as Texas attorney general (1886–1890), leader of the Texas Democratic Party (1887–1890), and governor of Texas (1890–1895). During that time, James cemented his reputation for stirring public addresses, which often advocated on behalf of "the little man" against big railroads, banks, and insurance companies.

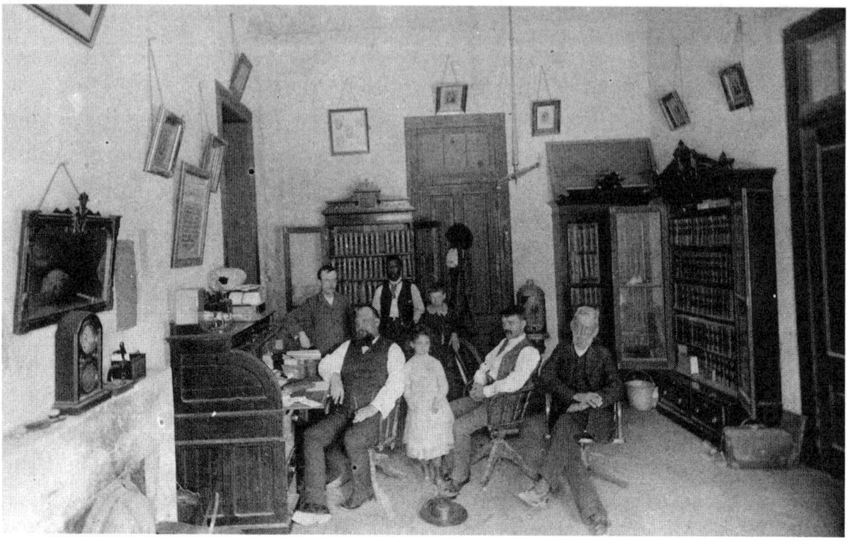

1.1. James Stephen Hogg (seated), Attorney General of Texas, at his desk in the Temporary Capitol at 11th Street and Congress Avenue, Austin, Texas, undated, c. 1887–91. Ima is standing behind James. Box 3T240–1. Ima Hogg Papers, Briscoe Center for American History, University of Texas at Austin.

In January 1891, when James was inaugurated as the first native-born Texan to be elected governor, his children Will (age sixteen) and Ima (age eight) attended his inauguration ceremony and ball. The family's tenure in the governor's mansion provided Ima with numerous experiences that would shape her worldview, including her approach to the Hogg Foundation much later. She observed political life at close range, learned to appreciate fine furnishings and antiques while helping her mother renovate the dilapidated mansion, took private music lessons from a German tutor, and traveled several times with her father on state business (including a trip to New York City).

Among these trips were numerous visits to the state's schools for children who were blind and deaf and state hospitals for adults and children who had been diagnosed with various types of mental illness. Mental health and illness had been interests of James Hogg for several years prior to his term as governor, but the extent of this interest is unclear. Hogg family profiles written many decades later suggest mental illness was a major concern. "Jim Hogg," one writer stated characteristically, "had great compassion for these individuals, and he read research on mental problems in hopes that one day they could be cured."[12] Indeed, the Hogg family library included several leading books on mental illness. But, preoccupied with reforms in the regulation of business and political lobbying, James did not place reform of the mental hospitals on his legislative agenda, nor does he appear to have spoken publicly about the subject. His concerns, in other words, were shared largely privately, and to a great extent with his daughter Ima, as would later be noted by Ima's biographers: "In Ima was born a special concern for those with mental illness who were lost inside those institutions."[13] In a 1970 interview, Ima recalled their shared visits with individual patients:

> I was also very much interested in mentally ill people in hospitals. . . . My father was very interested, also. . . . And often I went through with him and I'd hear him say to the superintendent or the doctor, "What can be done for these people? What are you doing?" And then I used to sit with them, many of them, and entertain them. I enjoyed talking with a lot of them, and they were all so homesick. They'd say they didn't belong there—their families sent them because they wanted to get rid of them . . . that was always in the wards where they weren't so mentally ill . . . they were disturbed people, melancholy people. I used to visit a great deal at the asylum. And I had little girl friends out there, you know, at the asylum where they had children. . . I was at the hospital all the time. . . . I was free to go into the wards any time I wanted to.[14]

These visits were cut short by a series of personal challenges that would provide Ima with a more intimate, if unplanned, introduction to mental health and mental illness. In 1895, just as James's final term of office concluded, Sallie's already fragile health took a turn for the worse when she was diagnosed with tuberculosis. That summer, Ima, at that time thirteen years old, accompanied her mother to a relative's home in Colorado, where it was hoped the dry air would improve her condition. Ima's mother tried to prepare Ima to take on a greater caregiving role for her younger brothers Mike and Tom while also urging her to pursue her education. With her family at her bedside, Sallie passed away on September 20, 1895. Sallie's death may have contributed to "periodic depressions" experienced by the youngest of the Hogg children, Tom, who was eight years old at that time. Later in life, Tom "wrestled with a drinking problem" and would have little involvement with the family business or the Hogg Foundation until his death in 1949.[15] For Ima, the death of her mother at the age of forty-one would be the first of several, including those of her father James Hogg (1906, age fifty-five), her older brother Will (1930, also age fifty-five), and her younger brothers Mike (1941, age fifty-six) and Tom (1949, age sixty-one). Ima would outlive them all by several decades, passing away in 1975 at the age of ninety-three years old.

One of Sallie's final directives to Ima was that she continue to pursue her education and that her education was equally as important as that of her brothers. Accordingly, Ima attended the University of Texas as a seventeen-year-old freshman in the fall of 1899. She would later recall that one of her favorite subjects was psychology, which she studied with Professor Caswell Ellis, a faculty member who later served on the first advisory council for the Hogg Foundation in 1940. In the fall of 1901, after two years at the university, Ima, then age nineteen, left to study piano and music at the National Conservatory of Music in New York City. Meanwhile, the family's economic fortunes had begun to take a dramatic turn for the better. James Hogg had become one of the early participants in the Texas oil boom that had begun with the Spindletop oil strike, near Beaumont in East Texas, in January 1901. That spring, James purchased 4,600 acres of adjacent land in nearby West Columbia and mineral rights to 15 acres on Spindletop hill in partnership with James Swayne, a friend and Fort Worth lawyer who had served in the legislature during James's governorship.[16] The partners formed the Hogg-Swayne Syndicate, which later became the Texas Company (Texaco). Even as James began to transform his new property, which included a former plantation, into a family home and farm, he continued to believe it contained oil reserves. This belief would be vindicated in 1917, when a large oil strike on the Varner property made the family extremely wealthy.[17]

In 1903 Ima returned from New York to take control of decorating and managing the family home at the Varner Plantation. As Ima transformed the old plantation into a gathering place for scattered family members, James gave up his law practice in Austin and opened a new one in Houston to be closer to home and to his booming new oil partnership. On a return trip from Houston in January 1905, James suffered a major neck injury in a train accident, one that would require several surgeries over the next year. On March 3, 1906, Ima entered James's bedroom to wake him from a nap for lunch, only to find that her father had died in his sleep of an apparent heart attack. Thus by the time she was only twenty-three years old, Ima had nursed both of her parents through debilitating illnesses and witnessed their deaths.

Encountering the Mental Hygiene Movement

According to his biographers, James Stephen Hogg had embraced mounting criticisms of large institutions and asylums for individuals with mental illness. In particular, Hogg subscribed to the notion that many forms of mental illness might be "cured" or ameliorated with medical, psychiatric, or psychological interventions that could allow individuals to live relatively normal lives outside of institutions. Generally, this reflected the Progressive Era belief that intractable problems of various kinds could be solved with the proper deployment of scientific expertise. However, "curing" mental illness presented a far different challenge than regulating railroad corporations or curtailing the influence of lobbyists in the state legislature. As we have seen, mental illness was poorly understood even by the experts of that era. However, a new national movement emerged in the first decades of the twentieth century, shortly after James's death. This movement, led by the National Committee for Mental Hygiene (NCMH), founded in 1909, promoted "mental hygiene" and advocated for community-based rather than institutional programs for persons living with mental illness. In the view of the NCMH, the nineteenth-century asylum not only failed to ameliorate "curable" conditions but often worsened them by imprisoning diagnosed individuals in custodial institutions. Members of the NCMH further argued that this regime stigmatized individuals who were perfectly capable of living in society, because mental "hygiene" and illness in their view occupied different locations on a shared continuum.[18] During the 1910s and 1920s, Ima Hogg would encounter the ideas and some of the key figures in this emerging movement due to her own struggles with depression. These experiences would lead Ima to resolve to bring mental health services and reforms to her home state of Texas.

After her father's death, Ima suffered a deep depression that was allayed by long visits to New York City (1906) and Europe (1907–9), where she immersed herself in the study of music. In fact, Ima's music studies culminated with her first significant philanthropic activity. In 1913 Ima helped organize the inaugural performance of the Houston Symphony and mounted fundraising and publicity campaigns to support its continuation. According to her biographers, Ima cultivated an attitude about the arts that was at once populist and avant-garde; she "composed dissonant music," purchased several pieces of then-controversial European modern art, and built a substantial collection of American Indian art. Later in her life, she sponsored music programs for less privileged children, often insisting that the symphony should belong to the masses as well as the classes. While this philosophy reflected the Hogg family's civic-mindedness, it also showed how that spirit helped to shape Ima's later approach to mental health. Like many modern women of her generation, Ima included the arts in her understanding of mental health; as she stated in an interview many years later, "anything that contributes to a wholesome life is mental health."[19]

Meanwhile, on January 15, 1918, a massive oil strike on the Varner plantation heralded the first of many such strikes and made the Hogg family into multimillionaires practically overnight. Will and Ima would become the driving forces behind the use of the money for philanthropic purposes, following in the spirit of their family's values. As virtually every biographer has noted, the Hogg children viewed themselves as "trustees" of the newfound family fortune, with a solemn responsibility to use it for the greater public good.[20] The family formed the Hogg Brothers company to manage the oil money responsibly. At the head of Hogg Brothers was Will, who, like his father, was physically imposing, personable, colorful, and generous.

Even as the family's fortunes changed, Ima's music-fueled respite from emotional distress came to an abrupt end during and shortly after World War I. Ima's brother Mike was wounded in action, and, shortly after that, Ima suffered a series of physical and emotional maladies, including a bout with the Spanish flu pandemic of 1918. Soon after, Ima experienced a five-year bout of "severe depression" that included a prolonged case of insomnia. Ima's doctors diagnosed her with "nervous exhaustion" and referred her to a neurologist in Philadelphia.[21] The vogue of psychoanalysis that had swept through the elite circles of several American cities largely had bypassed Texas, forcing Ima to seek treatment elsewhere. Between November 1923 and February 1924, Ima visited with the therapist Austin Fox Riggs at his clinic in Stockbridge, Massachusetts. A popular author and influential promoter of mental hygiene, Riggs introduced Ima to the concept of "positive mental health."[22] He also encouraged her to engage with the emerging national movement for mental hygiene, which in turn introduced Ima to the NCMH. Founder of the NCMH Clifford Beers, a former patient in the Massachusetts State Hospital, wrote about his experience in his influential book *The Mind That Found Itself* (1908).[23] The NCMH very quickly established itself as a force in the state of Texas and beyond. In its first decade of existence, the NCMH circulated a draft commitment law for individuals with mental illness that was adopted by several state legislatures, advocated for standards of treatment for mental hospitals and institutions, and conducted professional surveys of mental hospitals and clinical services for numerous states (including one for Texas completed in 1924). The NCMH also spread its message through state and local chapters; by 1920 the NCMH could claim at least one chapter in every state. In 1934 a group of 134 individuals, including Ima Hogg, met in the capitol building in Austin to form the Texas Society for Mental Hygiene.[24]

During this period, mental hygiene proponents such as Ima experimented with child guidance clinics in local communities. This special type of mental health clinic aimed to build on another Progressive Era reform—the juvenile court—which had been inaugurated in Chicago in 1899 and then spread across the nation (Houston was one of four Texas cities to adopt a juvenile court in 1907). This court was devised to prevent youthful offenders from becoming adult criminals by offering them treatment instead of punishment and by separating them from adults through community-based rehabilitation programs. Within a few years of the court's establishment, however, reformers came to feel that it did not intervene soon enough to prevent a delinquent and ultimately criminal career. This conviction gave birth to "child guidance," or the provision of outpatient clinical services for "pre-delinquent" children and their families prior to adolescence.[25] The prototypical clinic would be staffed with a team comprised of social workers, psychologists, and psychiatrists, who would collaborate to assess and devise interventions for what today would be called "at-risk" youth but at the time were labeled "problem children." In 1921 the Rockefeller Foundation's Commonwealth Fund partnered with the NCMH on the establishment of child guidance demonstration clinics in seven American cities over a five-year period, including one in Dallas founded in 1923. Ima learned of the Dallas clinic from Austin Riggs, who also showed Ima a child guidance clinic he was developing in Massachusetts. He encouraged Ima to research mental hygiene and child guidance and to develop a program for her home city of Houston.[26]

According to historians of the child guidance movement, these clinics attempted to offer many things at once, including prevention services through public education about mental hygiene for "normal" children and clinical treatment services for children with "adjustment" disorders. In many cases, the community education portion of the child guidance mission quickly dropped off, as clinics focused on providing treatment services for particular populations of children.[27] Indeed, the need for clinical services in Texas was becoming better understood by that time. In 1925, at the request of the Texas legislature, the NCMH conducted a statewide mental hygiene survey. Its final report called for more mental health clinics for children and adults, as well as more academic programs to train professionals who could staff clinics and hospitals.[28]

Ima's encounter with the NCMH and the child guidance movement also exposed her to the new brand of philanthropy that had emerged by the 1920s, as the historian Kate Sayen Kirkland has noted. The Rockefeller Foundation formed an umbrella organization of several large national philanthropies that embraced efficient management practices and targeted their funds strategically toward carefully researched social problems. In many cases, these problems had grown out of the social dislocations promulgated by industrialization, urbanization, and immigration during the late nineteenth and early twentieth centuries. Social science experts staffed these foundations, as well as government agencies, working to identify and devise solutions for these new social problems. According to Kirkland, by the time of the Hogg Foundation's creation in 1939–40, "a symbiotic public-private process had emerged: foundations and private institutions tried to influence social policy and government spending by identifying a need, financing and organizing pilot programs, garnering public enthusiasm, and then turning to government agencies for continued funding and maintenance."[29] This new paradigm for foundation work would greatly influence Ima's thinking about the Hogg Foundation, as well as her first foray into mental health philanthropy, the Houston Child Guidance Clinic.

On November 1, 1929, the Houston Child Guidance Clinic opened its doors at a rented house in central Houston, with a small staff that included a director and two social workers and a starting endowment of about $10,000.

This was less than half the annual budget of $25,000 estimated as minimally necessary by the founding board of directors. Similar concerns had been expressed by George Stevenson, director of Community Clinics for the Commonwealth Fund, who had visited Houston twice at Ima's request in 1926 and 1929.[30] Unable to procure support from the Commonwealth Fund, Ima nevertheless decided to rely on locally raised funds; however, this proved to be extremely challenging. Throughout the 1930s, the clinic struggled to stay afloat financially, forcing Ima to mount perpetual fundraising drives.[31] Prospects dimmed not only due to the Great Depression but because likely donors did not seem to share Ima's enthusiasm for, or understanding of, child guidance. Moreover, the clinic served poor and marginalized populations; about half of its initial referrals came from settlement homes, orphanages, and juvenile courts.[32] While this spoke well of the clinic's availability to all citizens, it also may have dampened donor enthusiasm. Ima remained on the clinic's board of directors for forty-six years and frequently provided funds either through personal donations or, later, through Hogg Foundation grants. The clinic would become more solvent in the 1940s, as the Houston Community Chest began providing significant annual funds, and, after 1948, the Texas Department of Health provided funds authorized under the National Mental Health Act.[33] Even as the Houston Child Guidance Clinic struggled through the 1930s, a new turn of events caused Ima to focus her attention on a larger mental health initiative, one that would be statewide in scope and that would be based at hers and her brother Will's alma mater, the University of Texas.

"The Cause That Would Live Up to the Hogg Family's Long-Held Ideals"

In September 1930 Will C. Hogg was enjoying the tenth month of a European vacation. His sister Ima had joined him at Baden-Baden, a health resort in Germany, when Will suddenly experienced a "gall bladder attack" and died abruptly on September 12 after emergency surgery at the age of fifty-five. Even as she accompanied her brother's body back to Texas, Ima began the process of thinking about "creating a memorial to Will" that would "live up to the Hogg family's long-held ideals of education and compassion."[34] Indeed, Will himself had set a particular kind of example in this area. As chair of the Board of Regents at the University of Texas in 1916–17, Will had clashed with Texas Governor James "Pa" Ferguson over university governance; Will had helped lead the campaign to have Ferguson impeached in 1917, citing his desire for a "university of the first class" that would serve the broader interests of Texas. A noted philanthropist throughout the 1920s, Will played a leading role in the creation of the University of Texas Ex-Students Associa-

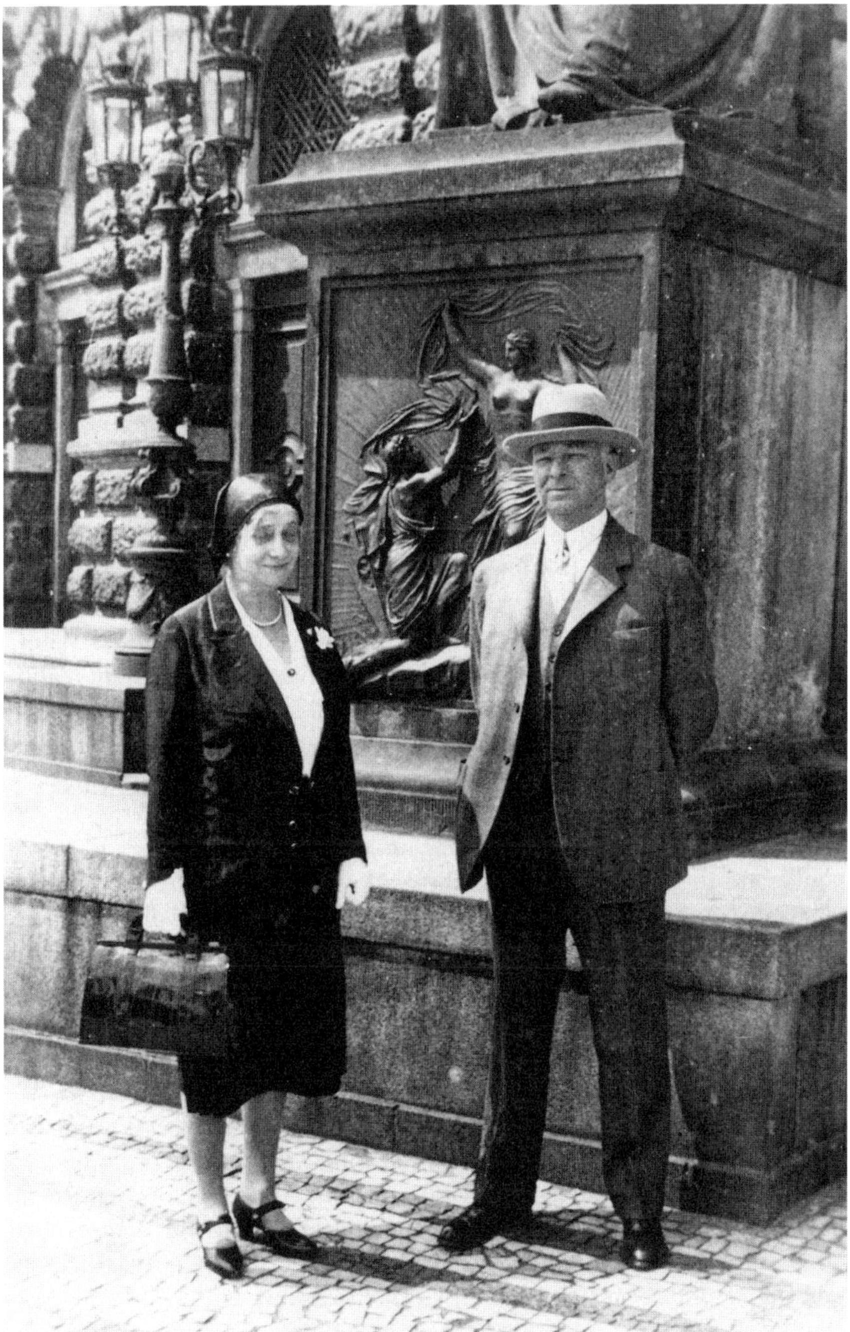

1.2. Ima and Will Hogg in Dresden, Germany, 1930, shortly before Will's death. Box 3T240–1. Ima Hogg Papers, Briscoe Center for American History, University of Texas at Austin.

tion and routinely encouraged his wealthy Houston-area friends to donate generously to various charitable causes. For his part, Will practiced what he preached, mostly behind the scenes, anonymously sponsoring tuition for promising but needy college students, particularly military veterans. In addition, Will quietly made donations to the University of Texas, Rice University, Texas A&M University, and Prairie View A&M University.[35]

After Will's death, it fell to his siblings Mike and Ima to dispose of his estate as stipulated in his will, which deeded about $2.5 million, nearly all of the estate's worth, to an endowment fund. The will spelled out three possible uses for the endowment: a vocational school for wayward boys and girls at Varner Plantation, a "Lecture Foundation" supervised by the Board of Regents of the University of Texas, or "any foundation or benefaction for the common good of all or any part of Texas to which either or both of them [Mike and Ima] may design to bequeath the bulk of their estate or estates."[36] Ima convinced her brother to dedicate the endowment to "the cause that would . . . live up to the Hogg family's long-held ideals."[37] After several months of negotiations, on July 15, 1939, the Will C. Hogg endowment was transferred to the Board of Regents of the University of Texas. The board was empowered to manage the endowment "in trust" for the wishes of Will C. Hogg as stated in his will.[38] Included in this arrangement was the stipulation that the endowment would be used for a mental health program, an activity that was neither specified nor suggested in the original Hogg will. However, the idea was a frequent topic of discussion between Ima and Will in the years prior to his unexpected death.

In fact, the will presented challenging legal obstacles for both the Hogg family and the university beyond the obvious absence of the words "mental health." Attorneys for both sides initially interpreted the will to limit the activities of a university-managed endowment to the lecture foundation specified as the second possible option. This meant that a purpose designated by Ima and Mike, as mentioned in the third option, could not be administered through the university. This conflict was resolved in 1938–39 after extended negotiations between attorneys for both sides and an investigation by a medical committee appointed by the Board of Regents resulted in a consensus that the proposed foundation could combine the two directives. But trouble resumed after Mike Hogg signed over the endowment to the university. Shortly after the public announcement of the transaction, Hogg family attorney Stephen Pinckney (who had participated in the negotiations) told the *Houston Post* that the transfer of the endowment to the university conflicted with Will's intentions just before his death to devote his personal fortune to civic projects for his home city of Houston—"which he considered the best place on earth."[39]

Even as the new foundation entered into its planning and early development stages, debate continued to rage behind the scenes over the question of what activities were permitted under the terms of the will. Some of the controversy reflected the uniqueness of the new arrangement; private foundations were still somewhat new devices in Texas, and the proposed Hogg Foundation would mark a number of firsts: the first professionally managed foundation in Texas, the first private foundation dedicated to the cause of mental health, and the first private foundation housed within a public university. The most serious internal objection came from the university's comptroller, J.W. Calhoun, who sent a five-page brief to President Rainey and at least one regent in the summer of 1940. Critical of "the universal assumption that this fund is an endowment for the study of mental hygiene," Calhoun contended that Ima and Mike Hogg's wishes "cannot change the conditions made by Will Hogg himself in his Will." The very act of transferring the Hogg endowment to the university meant that it could function only as a lecture foundation, as outlined in the second option of the will—a "mandate . . . not subject to debate or to comparison as to importance with any other enterprise." His language is worth quoting at length:

> What other conditions did Will Hogg attach to the use of his estate, what other suggestions did he make to the Regents as to the use of the funds? None, not another word. If one thing and only one thing was to be done with this money, what did Will Hogg want that thing to be? There can be no two opinions as to that if one gives the Will even the most casual reading. . . .
>
> If the terms of this Will, so far as it affects the Regents of the University of Texas, are not clear then surely no man can ever hope to state in unmistakable terms what he wishes done with money after he is no more. . . . There are but two courses open when money such as this is tendered to an institution. It must decline the offer or carry out the directions of the donor.[40]

Scarcely a year into its role as administrator of the Hogg endowment, the university thus found itself in the awkward position of debating donor intent with the donor's closest living relatives. The record suggests that an attempt was made to avoid a direct confrontation with Ima Hogg over the matter in 1940–42. Planning documents show that the Hogg Foundation's first director, Robert Sutherland, felt constrained by the mandate for educational lectureships, which limited his ability to carry out a mental hygiene program. At the same time, Sutherland asserted that mental hygiene was justified under the second option of the will:

> Since mental hygiene has come to be one of the most important subjects within the general area of social experience of mankind mentioned in the will, inasmuch as the Board of Regents has authority to designate the use

> of any residue of the funds not required in the other lectureships, and inasmuch as the executor and the sister of the deceased request that special emphasis be given this field, the Hogg Foundation director will present in broad and educational terms mankind's achievement in those phases of mental and social adjustment which are referred to by the term "mental hygiene."[41]

This formulation expressed well the rhetorical tightrope walked by the Hogg Foundation in these early years. Publicly, the Foundation equated its lectureships with its mental hygiene activities; privately, Sutherland and others felt caught between internal critics of these activities and Ima Hogg, who was not involved in this discussion and whose disapproval they feared should she become aware of it. The Foundation's first official stationery letterhead listed "Lectureships" ahead of "Mental Hygiene."[42] Invitation letters to the Foundation's three-day inaugural conference in February 1941 addressed "Texans Interested in Public Education and Mental Hygiene." "In addition to the lectureships," explained the invitation, "the Foundation will give major attention to the co-ordination and extension of mental hygiene services throughout the State."[43] In fact, the words "mental health" and "mental hygiene" did not appear prominently on either the tickets to the formal inaugural dinner or the cover of the conference's program booklet. This omission contrasted with the program's content, which included several conference panels focused explicitly on mental health. Although it was not exactly concealed, mental health nevertheless occupied a tentative place in the Foundation's overall program.

Several months earlier, in October 1940, Sutherland expressed concern that this state of affairs would not sit well with Ima Hogg. "With her present interpretation of the will," he confided to Rainey, "Miss Hogg may be very much surprised to see that the lectureship phase of the program is given prominence and that its scope is much broader than mental hygiene."[44] So concerned was Sutherland that he suggested a conference with the Hogg family and its attorneys, a move Rainey initially rejected. Sutherland's anxiety was allayed temporarily by Ima Hogg's positive reaction to the inaugural conference. However, the balancing act between educational lectureships and mental health activities continued, as evidenced by a description of the Foundation program in a letter written to Mike Hogg shortly before his death in October 1941. Here Sutherland listed "public education" as the top priority, citing "the specific request which appeared in your brother's will."[45]

It was only a matter of time before Ima became aware of the conflict. She explained her growing displeasure to Sutherland after the pair attended a Hogg Foundation–sponsored lecture in Houston. Confiding again to Rainey in March 1942, Sutherland wrote that "he was more convinced than ever that she will not be reassured concerning the interpretation of her brother's will until she receives an explanation in writing from the Board of Regents indicating that mental hygiene is to be the exclusive purpose of the Foundation."[46] Under sustained pressure from Sutherland, Rainey requested a formal evaluation from the University of Texas Land Attorney, who concluded that "a portion of this trust estate [Will's estate] can be used by the Board of Regents as a Lecture Foundation, and a portion thereof can be used in establishing and maintaining a mental health program as contemplated by Mr. Mike Hogg and Miss Ima Hogg."[47] This statement frustrated Ima Hogg, who desired that the Foundation that bore her family's name dispense with its divided program and focus all its energies on mental health. Ima sensed that her ambition for a far-reaching mental health program was in real jeopardy of becoming simply another program at the university, a fate she found intolerable. In a letter to Sutherland, Ima expressed this concern and issued a warning:

> As to the interpretation of my Brother's will . . . I can only say that the clause to which he refers (even if that alternative had been chosen by my Brother Mike and myself) if I remember rightly, indicated that "distinguished lecturers" be brought to Texas in the interest of broader education. It would hardly seem to me that my Brother Will meant to establish a fund to support a campaign or promotion office. My Brother Mike and I were perfectly clear as to our intentions when we finally decided upon a "Mental Health Foundation" for the University of Texas. And we believed we were clearly empowered to make that choice. . . .
>
> In my limited experience and observation, I find it is always difficult not to confuse issues. It is difficult to maintain a set aim single-mindedly—especially as the world is so full of crying needs and pressures. One might say that Mental Hygiene is not the most urgent cause in the world, but once having started on a program for its application—with all the manifold ramifications—one might find it ineffectual if repeated influences divert the effort from the main objective. The surface has hardly been touched in Texas.[48]

The disagreement culminated in an official report, written by President Rainey and presented to the Board of Regents at their meeting of October 23, 1942. The Rainey report argued that the Foundation combined two of the three potential directives laid out in the Hogg will and that this was permissible. According to the report, the second option enabled the endowment's transfer to the university, while the third option allowed Mike and Ima Hogg to create "any foundation or benefaction for the common good of all or any part of Texas." In addition, the report conveyed a warning from Ima: "She has

. . . instructed me to say to the Board of Regents that unless it is clearly understood that her brother's estate is to be used for a mental hygiene foundation, she and other members of her family will no longer feel under obligation to turn their estates into the Foundation."[49] In response, the board appointed a special subcommittee to investigate the matter. A report was presented to the board at its January 8, 1943, meeting, recommending that the board agree upon the name "Hogg Foundation for Mental Hygiene," which it did by unanimous vote.[50]

Even before this final disagreement played itself out, President Rainey and Ima Hogg had begun the work of articulating the Foundation's mental hygiene mission. Equally as critically, this new mission needed to be commensurate with a limited operating budget. The Foundation's annual budget would draw upon proceeds from the endowment's investment earnings rather than directly from the endowment itself. In its first year (1940–41), the Foundation's operating budget amounted to about $32,000; it would remain around that amount during its first decade, falling as low as $21,000 at times.[51] This reality meant that another important decision for Rainey and Ima would be the recruitment and identification of a leader for the new Foundation who could maximize its limited financial resources and perhaps even attract additional support.

"A Mental Health Program for the People of Texas"

A terse statement of the Foundation's mission appeared in the legal agreement transferring the Hogg endowment to the Board of Regents on July 15, 1939. The endowment would provide a "fund" for a "mental health program" for "the people of Texas," which the Hogg family felt "could be best done through the University of Texas."[52] Both President Rainey and Ima Hogg believed that they would need to seek out expert advice to transform that broad imperative into a more specific plan of action. Together, they formed an advisory committee to assist with defining the Foundation's mission further and leading a national search for a director. In addition to Ima and President Rainey, the committee included some of the nation's top experts in mental health: Dr. George Stevenson, medical director of the National Committee for Mental Hygiene; Dr. Daniel Prescott of the University of Chicago Psychology Department; and Dr. Adolph Meyer, who headed both the NCMH and the Psychiatry Department at the Johns Hopkins University Medical School. Through her communications with the Commonwealth Fund and the NCMH, Ima had met each of these individuals and had personally invited them to join the advisory committee.[53] The committee convened for a two-day meeting at the University of Texas on January 29 and 30, 1940, which by all accounts was a model of collaboration between individuals from various backgrounds and perspectives on mental health. Meyer, who dined with Ima in Houston to discuss the Foundation one-on-one, expressed this sentiment shortly after the committee meeting in a letter to Ima: "[Mental health] is one of those movements in which the trained scientist and the intelligent and wholehearted layman have to work hand in hand."[54] After the advisory meeting, Daniel Prescott described Ima as "a person of extraordinary culture, common sense, and insight... [who will] turn out to be of great help in ways other than financial to the person who directs the foundation."[55] So enthused was the NCMH that its board of directors elected Ima to full membership as "an acknowledgement and recognition of the professional and lay persons active in fields related to mental hygiene."[56] The advisory committee's final report issued five specific recommendations: (a) survey mental health conditions in Texas, (b) establish mental health clinics across the state, (c) provide mental health instruction in Texas teacher-training courses, (d) provide facilities for mental health research at the University of Texas School of Medicine, and (e) promote mental health lectures at the University of Texas and across the state.[57] All but the final item were shelved initially due to limited funds and concerns about the donor's desire for lectureships.[58] During the Foundation's first decade, its mission would consist of a combination of components (c) and (e). The Foundation sponsored public lectures across the state as well as at the University of Texas; delivered consultation services to assist local professionals in setting up mental health services in existing institutions such as schools or stand-alone mental health clinics; reprinted mental health lectures, essays, and articles in pamphlets distributed to a growing mailing list; advocated for new and reformed academic programs to train professionals in the disciplines most closely related to mental health; and cosponsored in-service training seminars on mental health for professionals in a variety of fields. One point of emphasis for the advisory committee was that the Foundation should avoid much direct involvement with the state's mental hospitals; instead, the Foundation should engage in public educational activities and emphasize mental health needs outside of institutions. In fact, as we shall see in chapter 3, the Foundation would not be able to avoid involvement with Texas' system of mental hospitals.

Enthusiasm continued to run high in the wake of the advisory committee meeting. "If you had Barnum-blood in your veins," joked Evelyn Carrington, secretary for the Texas Society for Mental Hygiene, "you would have made us pay an admission to hear Dr. Meyer, Dr. Stevenson and Dr. Prescott."[59] This spilled over into the next important task, which fell largely to President Rainey, "to find an outstanding director for this problem, and then leave the program largely to his own understanding and initiative."[60] Armed with several recommendations from the advisory committee, Rainey began the search. The short list provided to Rainey included John Rose, director of the Philadelphia Child Guidance Clinic; George E. Gardner, a fellow at the Judge Baker Child Guidance Center in Boston; and James P. Molloy Jr., director of the Houston Child Guidance Clinic.[61] However, Rainey seems to have decided that the position called for someone with a "broader social science" background, less tied to the fields most closely associated with mental hospitals and comfortable both inside and outside the academy. Therefore, Rainey reached out to one of his longtime colleagues, Robert Lee Sutherland, who Rainey had known for "nine years in a very intimate way," as he later explained to Ima.[62] At the time, Sutherland held several positions: chair of the Social Sciences Department at Bucknell University in Pennsylvania, a position he had held for nearly a decade; Associate Vice-President and Dean of Men, a position he had held for four years; and Associate Director of the American Youth Commission, based on Washington, DC. In April 1940 Sutherland visited Austin to meet with Rainey, Ima, and individual members of the Board of Regents, all of whom concluded that Sutherland was the right choice for the directorship. Sutherland opted to accept the directorship over offers for presidential appointments at two other universities.[63] The Hogg Foundation appealed to Sutherland, he later explained, because it offered him "a field where new projects can be started" rather than "general administrative work of a more traditional type."[64]

The close personal and professional relationship between Rainey and Sutherland surely aided in that decision. Both were graduate alumni from the storied sociology program at the University of Chicago, where Sutherland had earned a doctoral degree in 1930 after completing his dissertation, an ethnographic study of the African American churches on Chicago's south side. When Sutherland was hired as a professor of sociology at Bucknell University, his department chair was none other than Homer Rainey. Sutherland's career blossomed at Bucknell. He was the lead author of a textbook, *Introductory Sociology* (1935), which was in use at 250 colleges and universities at the time he accepted the Hogg Foundation directorship and which would go through seven editions. When the Rockefeller Foundation's American Council on Education established a five-year research program on American youth—the American Youth Commission (AYC)—Rainey was appointed as the director and Sutherland as an associate director supervising the AYC's "Negro Project."[65] In recommending his former protégé, Rainey highlighted his interpersonal, administrative, and public relations skills, all critical needs because mental health and its implications were virtually unknown in Texas.[66]

These skills had been honed during Sutherland's administration of the AYC's Negro Project, which began early in 1938 and produced four major book-length studies of African American youth in different parts of the United States.[67] Each book in the AYC monograph series presented lengthy life histories of individual black teenagers from different class backgrounds,

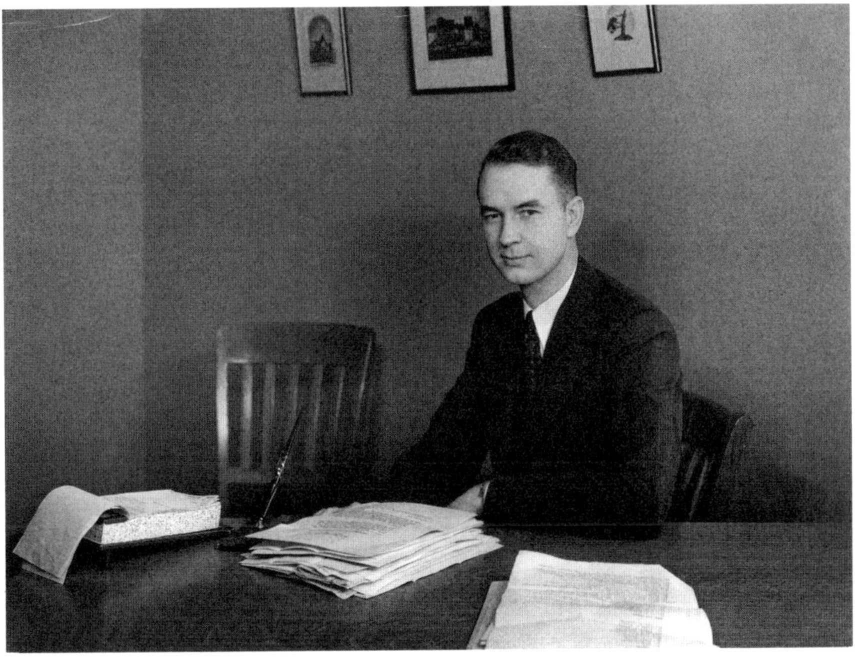

1.3. Robert Lee Sutherland in his office, undated, c. early 1940s. Box 2AA52B, Hogg Foundation for Mental Health Collection, Briscoe Center for American History, University of Texas at Austin.

drawn largely from interviews, field notes, and regional social survey data.[68] The researchers' shared hypothesis held that racism inflicted its worst psychological damage during childhood and adolescence. Sutherland underscored this thesis emphatically in his summary of the AYC studies, titled *Color, Class, and Personality*. "From his earliest days," he noted, "[the black child] is made to feel different and often inferior."[69] In this project, Sutherland adopted a presentation style that combined detached scholarship, a quasi-religious sense of mission, and reform-minded advocacy, an approach he would refine effectively in his subsequent role as director of the Hogg Foundation.

Sutherland's contemporaries would later cite these qualities in their recollections, portraying both a skilled diplomat and an unconventionally down-to-earth intellectual. Potential adversaries found themselves quickly disarmed by his "folksy" and "friendly" manner. A typical day for Sutherland began before dawn with a visit to Maudie's Cafe, where he would pore over notes from various ongoing research projects. Immediately after sunrise, Sutherland would "wander up the Low Water Bridge, and he'd stay on Redbud [Trail] till he got up to the top of the circle, way at the top." This location was dubbed "The Hill," an acre of forest he had purchased in west Austin—"a pretty good sized hill, almost a mountain." There Sutherland would dictate and write in a small work space—a "little cement block house" that he had built himself. "[B]y 10:00 he'd be done and he'd take it down and give it to his secretary." Lengthy discussions with colleagues on the issues of the day took place while Sutherland cooked bacon and eggs over a campfire. Sutherland's somewhat bohemian routine meshed well with the laid-back atmosphere of Austin, and his relaxed demeanor proved "able to interact with all kinds."[70]

These qualities stemmed from Sutherland's eclectic upbringing. Born in the rural town of Clarinda, Iowa, to attorney Donald Grant Sutherland and his wife Charlotte in 1903, Sutherland moved to Seattle, Washington, at the age of two and then to Galesburg, Illinois, at the age of fifteen. Sutherland would later tell people that he "financed [his] way through high school" in Galesburg by "raising pure bred livestock."[71] He attended Knox College in Illinois, earning a bachelor's degree in sociology in 1925. After teaching public speaking at a small college for a year, Sutherland completed a master's degree in theology at the socially progressive Oberlin College in 1927, where he wrote a thesis titled "Relation Between Eschatology and Jesus' Ethics," which attempted to demonstrate the ethical lessons offered by the historical Jesus.[72] The influence of religious belief continued in Sutherland's dissertation, a field study of African American churches in Chicago, which resulted in his doctoral degree being awarded in the field of Christian theology and ethics. A quiet determination and sense of mission would infuse Sutherland's leadership style at the Hogg Foundation; although low key in his personal mannerisms, Sutherland exerted a subtle kind of moral suasion over the various public officials, academic administrators, wealthy donors, mental health professionals, and lay citizens with whom he interacted comfortably on a daily basis. As his colleague Ira Iscoe later recalled, Sutherland was "most temperate . . . [and] never raised his voice. On the other hand, you never wished to disappoint Bob Sutherland."[73] Sutherland excelled at inspiring his staff and colleagues to persevere through difficult circumstances, particularly in the Foundation's early lean years. "Circuit riders," a label that Sutherland concocted, was only in part his tongue-in-cheek way to describe his and the Foundation's work in the 1940s, a project to which we turn next.

2

Spreading the Gospel of Mental Health in the 1940s and 1950s

During the first week of September 1952, a Hogg Foundation consultant named Joseph H. Lumpkin Jr. delivered a series of lectures on group and individual counseling to an audience of African American schoolteachers in Palestine, Texas. A small town that served as a railroad hub in east central Texas, Palestine organized its population of about 13,000 according to the Jim Crow system of racial segregation that predominated through much of the South as well as some other parts of the country.[1] Accordingly, Lumpkin had delivered separate lectures to an all-white audience of teachers prior to visiting with the region's black teachers. A doctoral student in the Education Department at the University of Texas at Austin, Lumpkin had spoken to many groups before, but he received a different kind of reception after this particular lecture.[2] He described the response in a memo to Hogg Foundation director Robert Sutherland:

> One elderly negro teacher asked for recognition from the superintendent after I had finished speaking and said something to this effect: "I not only want to express my personal thanks to this speaker this morning, but to the Hogg Foundation for sending him to us. I feel like I know Mr. Jim Hogg, I've heard about how he helped people in Texas while he was living. And some folks have a way of continuing to serve their people even after they're gone. Mr. Hogg's family, Miss Ima and the rest, have seen to that through this Hogg Foundation. I feel like Mr. Hogg is still serving folks in Texas this morning." My memory does not recall all her sincere eloquence, but that is a fair representation of what she said.[3]

As this anecdote suggests, the Foundation from the outset went out of its way to include diverse populations in its mental health outreach efforts. As we shall see, the Foundation sometimes did so even over the objections of local whites, with effects that were sometimes hard to gauge. Less in doubt was the scope of the Hogg Foundation's enterprise, which sought to reach as many people, and as many different groups of people, as possible around the state. Palestine was one of three Foundation-sponsored stops that year for Lumpkin, who also provided consulting services to the Lubbock Council of Churches and the Texas State Teachers' Association.[4] And Lumpkin was but one of many experts dispatched by the Foundation around the state's 254 counties. In its first three years alone, the Hogg Foundation sent lecturers and consultants to address some 2,000 audiences in 152 communities, reaching roughly 400,000 people. This number included talks or seminars at 40 colleges and 70 elementary or high schools. These events provided some of the material for a pamphlet series titled "Lectures in Print," which also reprinted scholarly articles and long-form journalistic accounts of mental health stories, in addition to Foundation-sponsored lectures. By October 1943, the Foundation had published 33 pamphlets and more than 49,000 separate pieces of mailed literature; by 1953 its mailing list exceeded 2,600. Foundation staff conducted in-service trainings with public education staff in urban and rural areas and with social workers and case workers in larger cities and helped devise a mental health program for medical students at the University of Texas medical branch in Galveston.[5]

Like Lumpkin, most of the Foundation's speakers were not full-time staff but rather had been hired on an ad hoc consulting basis. As noted in chapter 1, however, the Foundation's financial resources in these early years only went so far in supporting expert consultant fees and honorariums. Director Sutherland utilized an extensive network of professional connections to bring nationally known speakers such as Margaret Mead, as well as regional experts, for miniature speaking tours at reasonable prices. But even these opportunities were too limited to meet the perceived statewide demand for mental health education, awareness, and programming. Therefore the relatively small in-house staff spent much of its time traveling around the state delivering lectures and leading workshops—sometimes visiting several locations in a single day. During his first three years as Foundation director, Robert Sutherland himself gave 460 lectures in 56 different communities, returning to some places several times.[6] Sutherland was joined by a small group of energetic individuals with diverse academic and professional backgrounds to carry out the outreach program, many of whom were considered "staff" even though their paid appointment was funded either through a department of the University of Texas or a state agency.

The earliest such staff member was Bernice "Bunk" Milburn Moore (1904–1992), who joined the Hogg Foundation in 1944 and would remain there for twenty years while also serving as a consultant to the Texas Education Agency's Division of Home and Family Life Education.[7] A native of San Antonio and a graduate of the University of Texas, where she earned

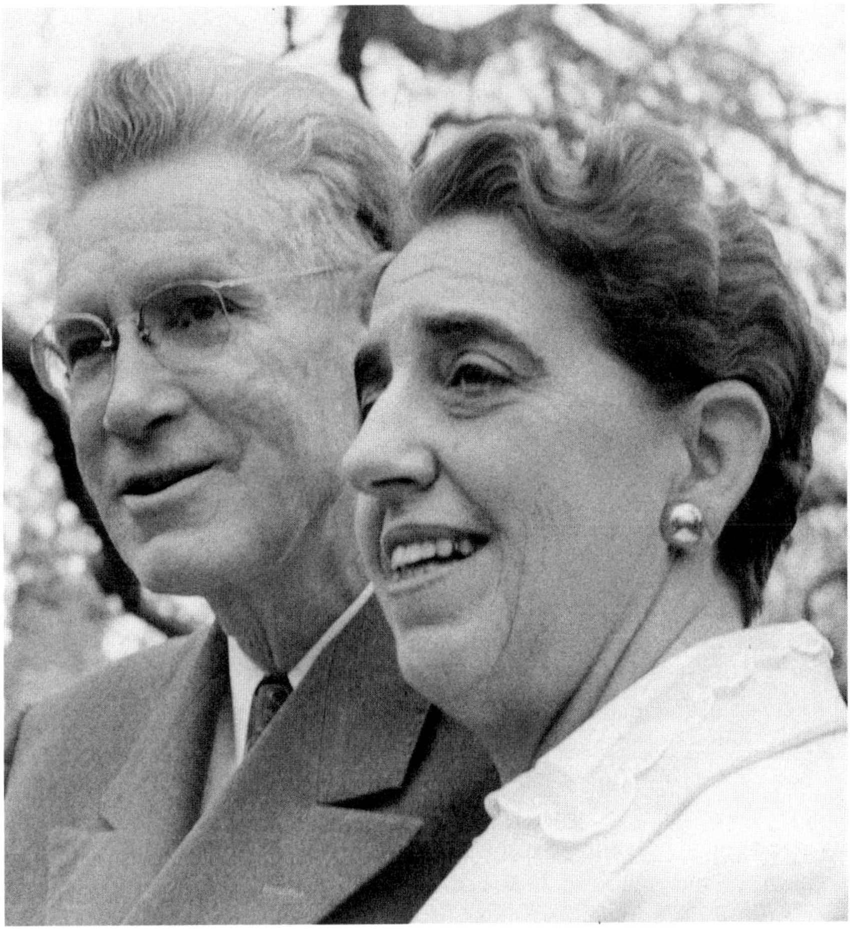

2.1. Bernice Milburn and Harry Estill Moore, undated. Box 98–285–15, Hogg Foundation Papers. Courtesy of the Briscoe Center for American History, University of Texas at Austin.

bachelor's and master's degrees in journalism, Moore took a somewhat circuitous route to the Foundation. During her graduate studies, she met her future husband Harry Estill Moore; after working in the newspaper business for a few years the pair migrated to the University of North Carolina at Chapel Hill, where they completed doctoral degrees in sociology and rural economics (Bernice) and sociology (Harry). In 1937 they returned to the University of Texas, where Harry began a tenure-track faculty appointment in the sociology department. The available evidence suggests Bernice was a forceful, outgoing personality; her nickname, Bunk, came from her time as a jazz musician. In a 1939 biographical statement, she described herself as follows: "I have Malta Fever and am as mean as hell, am 34 goin' on 35, and weigh 145 pounds and adore my husband and anything else you want to say."[8] Bernice took on a leading role in the Foundation's speaker series on women and families in the 1940s and conducted numerous family life studies for the Foundation in subsequent decades, as we shall see. She was a core figure in the Foundation's early history.

The speakers group followed Sutherland's lead in approaching their work with a quasi-religious sense of mission. Its members came to view themselves, in a phrase coined by Sutherland, as "circuit riders for mental health," driving the Texas highways and farm-to-market roads to bring the gospel of mental health to people who seldom received visitors from outside their town or county. "A new type of circuit rider visits Texas families today," announced the *DeLeon Free Press* in January 1948.[9] The Foundation's own publications began employing the phrase regularly, and it quickly entered the organization's mythology. A 1973 pamphlet gives a characteristic retrospective on the Foundation's early years, noting that most Texans had never heard the phrases "mental hygiene," "mental health," or "mental illness." In response, "a new type of circuit rider came upon the scene," and a host of Foundation experts "began an endless trek across the thousands of miles of Texas."[10] Longtime Foundation administrator Wayne Holtzman later recalled the genesis of the nickname:

> Bob [Sutherland] came from a family where there were ministers. I did too. And so a circuit rider seemed like a familiar term that would be kind of easy to use. And it did imply that you went out on a circuit. You went out to this town and that town and the next town, and you might spend lunch at one place, breakfast at another, dinner at another. And you'd have a round for a day or two that way, and then you'd come back to home base and go out again later. So in between classes I was partly a circuit rider, along with Bob Sutherland, Bernice Moore, and Bert [Kruger Smith], by that time not only a journalist but also a knowledgeable person to talk about mental health.[11]

This whirlwind of activity coincided with, and benefited from, historic transformations in the field of mental health. The national mobilization of resources promulgated by the outbreak of World War II included psychiatrists, psychologists, social scientists, and social workers. Psychiatrists in particular helped devise protocols for the screening of draftees and the treatment of soldiers traumatized by prolonged exposure to combat environments. These experiences, as the historian of psychiatry Gerald N. Grob has described, lent a new legitimacy to long-standing claims of the mental hygiene movement about the nature of, and appropriate approaches to, mental health and illness.[12] Soldiers who passed psychiatric draft screening protocols but who exhibited neurotic disorders under combat stress provided powerful support to the continuum theory of mental health and illness, which held that even "normal" individuals could experience mental disorders under certain conditions. Army psychiatrists devised preventive measures, most notably limited tour rotations to balance periods of protracted combat with periods of respite. The success of such measures, which sharply reduced combat-induced psychological discharges, suggested that prevention techniques could also be useful in civilian settings. Similarly, the development of successful treatments in the field rather than the hospital bolstered long-standing claims for the effectiveness of mental health treatment provided outside of institutional settings. Led by William Menninger, the first psychiatrist to achieve the rank of brigadier general, wartime psychiatrists forcefully argued that the lessons learned during the war could be applied to postwar society. Menninger led a faction of psychiatrists within the American Psychiatric Association in arguing further that the mental health professions should increasingly view the community rather than the hospital as their primary workplace. In his influential 1948 book *Psychiatry in a Troubled World: Yesterday's War and Tomorrow's Challenges*, Menninger envisioned the provision of war-developed mental health innovations in industrial workplaces, white-collar offices, criminal justice programs, public schools, and other everyday family and community settings. "The lessons we have learned in the combat zone," enthused two of Menninger's colleagues, "can well be applied in rehabilitation at home."[13]

Punctuating these shifts in the postwar era was the growing role of the federal government in mental health generally and community-based mental health particularly. The passage of the National Mental Health Act in 1946 and subsequent formation of the National Institute of Mental Health (NIMH) in 1949 established a major institutional base for the national mental health movement. Led by psychiatrist Robert Felix who, along with Menninger, would serve on the Hogg Foundation's national advisory board in the postwar era, the NIMH funded grants-in-aid explicitly for community-based mental health services rather than mental hospitals. This emphasis came at a time when those old-line institutions were coming under renewed criticism (see chapter 3). The NIMH also promoted the inclusion of "non-medical" experts such as social and behavioral scientists in the design and provision of mental health services—an interdisciplinary outlook that would form a major part of the Hogg Foundation's approach to mental health.

Swept up in these shifting winds, the Hogg Foundation worked closely with the military authorities in Texas during the war years while also educating all manner of public audiences about the myriad ways in which mental health promised to improve their lives. As a result, the Foundation found itself at the center of a host of social changes.

"Positive Mental Health in War-Time"

The American entry into World War II in December 1941 had a galvanizing effect on Texas' elected officials and its populace. With 5 percent of the nation's population, Texas provided 7 percent of the personnel who served in the armed forces. Of the 750,000 who served, including 12,000 women, the Texas contingent suffered a little over 22,000 casualties. While state and federal authorities mobilized military personnel, the agricultural and manufacturing sectors expanded their productive capacities to meet increased needs for food, fuel, synthetic rubber, steel, paper products, aircraft, and ammunition. Amid this increased demand, employers faced a labor shortage with most able young men joining the armed forces. The result was a workforce comprised substantially of younger people, nonwhites, and women, as well as a dramatic series of internal migrations to Texas' metropolitan areas. Partly as a result of this, the decade of the 1940s witnessed the transition of Texas from a predominantly rural to an urban state.[14] The onset of war, coupled with rapid social, economic, and demographic changes, provided the Hogg Foundation with numerous war-related demands for its services. The word "adjustment" became something of a mantra for the fields of psychiatry and psychology during and after the war. Mental health professionals assisted soldiers in coping with the rigors of combat and families and civilians adapting to the stresses of relocation and with absent, maimed, or deceased loved ones. Toward the end of the war, experts began to develop programs to assist returning veterans in adjusting to civilian life (it is no accident that the official name of the 1944 GI Bill was the Serviceman's *Readjustment* Act, or that it included funding for clinical psychological and psychiatric services).[15]

One of the first wartime requests made of the Hogg Foundation stemmed from the screening process for military draftees. In early 1942, the Foundation was contacted by Lt. Col. Franklin G. Ebaugh, neuropsychiatric consultant for the Eighth Service Command, headquartered in Dallas. A professor in the School of Medicine at the University of Colorado, Ebaugh had been an early proponent of "community-oriented psychiatry." One of his students, Robert Felix, would go on to lead the NIMH in the postwar era.[16] At the war's outset, the draft screening process consisted only of "a few minutes interview" between a military psychiatrist and an inductee, with little prior information about individual inductees provided to the induction staff. In response, Ebaugh advised the medical director of the state's Selective Service agency to work with the Hogg Foundation to develop "a demonstration procedure whereby social and health histories of selectees could be made available to the examining psychiatrists in the Induction Centers."[17] The initial psychiatric screening interview had done little to prevent an "unnecessarily large" number of discharges for "mental and emotional breakdowns," giving rise to the desire for a more robust screening process.[18] Coordinated by the Hogg Foundation—with director Sutherland named advisor to the state Selective Service director—this "Medical Survey Project" thus aimed to provide induction boards with educational, health, and criminal justice records prior to the induction interview.[19] The project proved to be daunting in scope, particularly after it was discovered that the Texas Department of Public Welfare, the state agency nominally tasked with compiling "social and health histories," had failed to do so due to a lack of adequate numbers of "medical field agents." The Foundation attempted to fill this void, asking its five-member staff to serve as a liaison between 254 county governments and the state's Selective Service board in gathering the records. In August 1945, Sutherland openly complained about the "tremendous amount of work" he and his staff had put forth merely to collect thousands of educational records (they were unable to procure health or psychological records).[20] The Foundation also provided other services to the Eighth Service Command, including advice manuals for the psychiatric screening of inductees and seminars for military chaplains on the provision of "preventive counseling" to stressed soldiers.[21] Toward the war's end, the Foundation announced that chaplains trained in counseling had reduced the number of psychiatric discharges at Fort Hood by more than 50 percent.[22]

Despite these strains, the Foundation agreed to a second request from the Eighth Service Command to conduct a study of Texas soldiers who had been discharged for "neuropsychiatric reasons." Sutherland assigned this study to Beulah Temple Wild, a psychiatric social worker trained at the University of Chicago, who was then working at the Houston Bureau of Mental Hygiene (formerly the Houston Child Guidance Clinic; see chapter 1). Wild already had joined the Foundation's stable of expert consultants, having been "loaned to the El Paso schools" for extended workshops with guidance counselors and teachers in the spring of 1941.[23] She produced a sample study of 211 discharged soldiers from five major Texas cities that included "brief case summaries . . . on men who had a history of mental illness or of maladjustment in their community and employment relations" prior to enlistment.[24] Wild met with the soldiers at the Bureau of Mental Hygiene in Houston; the Child Guidance Clinic had broadened its mission to meet wartime needs and had begun to serve veterans and their families as well. The study revealed two categories within the sample group: soldiers who passed the screening process despite a history of mental illness and soldiers without such a history who nevertheless began exhibiting emotional distress during or after combat situations. Wild's conclusion, echoing those of military psychiatrists, was that mental health services were needed in the field for military personnel and in the community for both veterans and civilians.

Amplifying these conclusions were a series of lectures and consulting sessions held across Texas to help "combat hysteria and war nerves" on the home front.[25] In his travels around the state shortly after the attack on Pearl Harbor, Sutherland found that adult citizens were "learning to hate each other" while children were "learning to hate" enemy populations, particularly the Japanese.[26] He urged audiences to "hate a bad system of control but not a fourth of the world's population" and to find "purposeful activities" that could focus anxieties productively.[27] "This is proof," he noted to a reporter for the *Austin Statesman*, "of the need for positive mental health in the nation during wartime."[28] Sutherland urged audiences of civic leaders, educators, and employers to encourage their communities to pull together for the war effort while resisting the urge to engage in negative behavior.[29] During the war years, Foundation consultants visited 70 high schools to discuss "wartime problems of adjustment" with teachers as well as students.[30]

At the same time, the Foundation provided female speakers to address audiences of women on how best to adjust to their changing roles during the war. Perhaps the best-known such speaker was Margaret Mead, the cultural anthropologist who had gained national recognition for her study of Samoan adolescent girls and wrote widely on women's roles in modern society (see Figure 2.2). Another speaker, Alice McConnell, was a supervisor for women trainees in aircraft repair as well as a "counselor for women in war for the Hogg Foundation."[31] Meanwhile, Bernice Milburn Moore lectured before more genteel and largely female audiences such as local chapters of the Parent-Teacher Association or the Rotary Club. One such lecture, titled "The Changing Family in the Changing World," urged working women to embrace their newfound opportunities while maintaining traditional household and childrearing duties.[32] Foundation speakers occasionally highlighted the expanded opportunities afforded to women by the war. "The Women's Army Corps has helped destroy the final tabu [sic], assuring an equal status for women in the post-war world," Sutherland declared in one talk, going further:

> The Women's Army Corps has helped remove the few lingering superstitions about the efficiency of women workers. When, during wartime, women can replace men in important types of military work, their ability to be trained for almost any type of service is established. . . . Women have an important place in the home, women have an important place in business and industry, and now women have an important status in our military organization. All of this development should lead to the more complete acceptance of women in the task of post-war planning. In the future, conference tables will have men and women working together planning the solution of international problems, as well as home front affairs.[33]

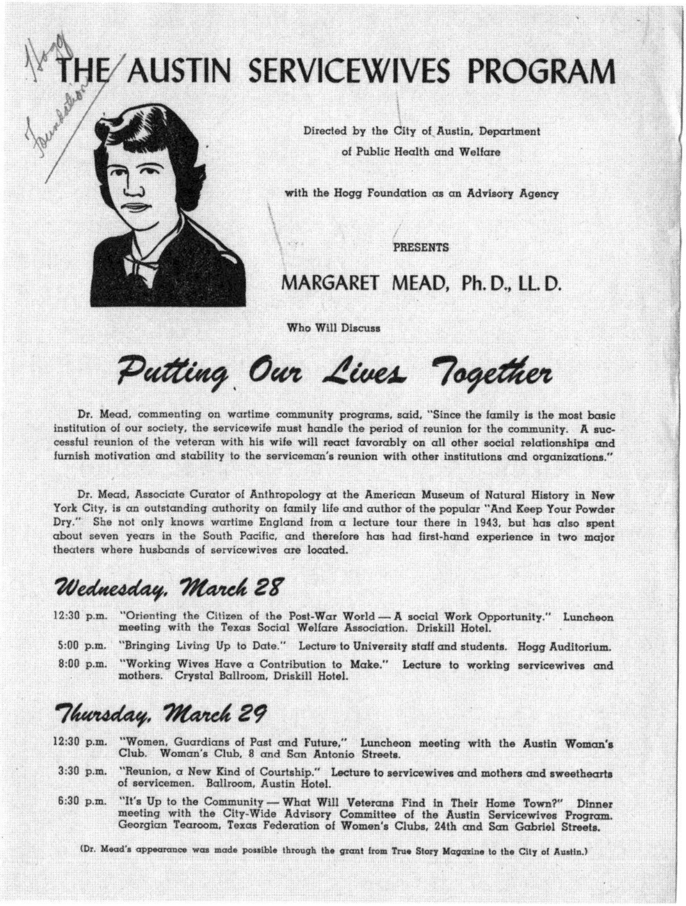
THE AUSTIN SERVICEWIVES PROGRAM

Directed by the City of Austin, Department of Public Health and Welfare

with the Hogg Foundation as an Advisory Agency

PRESENTS

MARGARET MEAD, Ph. D., LL. D.

Who Will Discuss

Putting Our Lives Together

Dr. Mead, commenting on wartime community programs, said, "Since the family is the most basic institution of our society, the servicewife must handle the period of reunion for the community. A successful reunion of the veteran with his wife will react favorably on all other social relationships and furnish motivation and stability to the serviceman's reunion with other institutions and organizations."

Dr. Mead, Associate Curator of Anthropology at the American Museum of Natural History in New York City, is an outstanding authority on family life and author of the popular "And Keep Your Powder Dry." She not only knows wartime England from a lecture tour there in 1943, but has also spent about seven years in the South Pacific, and therefore has had first-hand experience in two major theaters where husbands of servicewives are located.

Wednesday, March 28

12:30 p.m. "Orienting the Citizen of the Post-War World — A social Work Opportunity." Luncheon meeting with the Texas Social Welfare Association. Driskill Hotel.

5:00 p.m. "Bringing Living Up to Date." Lecture to University staff and students. Hogg Auditorium.

8:00 p.m. "Working Wives Have a Contribution to Make." Lecture to working servicewives and mothers. Crystal Ballroom, Driskill Hotel.

Thursday, March 29

12:30 p.m. "Women, Guardians of Past and Future." Luncheon meeting with the Austin Woman's Club. Woman's Club, 8 and San Antonio Streets.

3:30 p.m. "Reunion, a New Kind of Courtship." Lecture to servicewives and mothers and sweethearts of servicemen. Ballroom, Austin Hotel.

6:30 p.m. "It's Up to the Community — What Will Veterans Find in Their Home Town?" Dinner meeting with the City-Wide Advisory Committee of the Austin Servicewives Program. Georgian Tearoom, Texas Federation of Women's Clubs, 24th and San Gabriel Streets.

(Dr. Mead's appearance was made possible through the grant from True Story Magazine to the City of Austin.)

2.2. Margaret Mead flyer, 1943. Box 1991/016–58, Chairmen Lanning, Logan, Ashley, and Baker files, Texas State Board of Control Board members files, Archives and Information Services Division, Texas State Library and Archives Commission.

Sometimes the audiences included both lay and professional participants, as in a three-day workshop hosted in Dallas titled "Guidance for Youth in a World at War," which was offered to "teachers, counselors, group workers, service club members, and parents."[34] To lead the workshop, the Foundation brought in the director of guidance counseling from the New Rochelle, New York, public school district. Sessions were organized around a fictional adolescent character named "Johnny Jones" and focused on how best to foment "healthy" experiences in the classroom, in the home, and with peers. In fact, the Foundation devoted much of its "home front mental health" activities to the problems of children and youth. Even a March 1942 conference ostensibly dedicated to the issue of adult education showed this heightened focus. Cosponsored by the Hogg Foundation and the University of Texas Extension Center, the conference concluded with a lecture on "The Morale of Youth in a Time of War."[35] Attendees came from all over the state, including Tyler, Crockett, Corpus Christi, Lytle, Laredo, College Station, Mexia, San Antonio, Dallas, Orange, Godley, Bastrop, and Wichita Falls. Of particular concern for educators was the rising high school dropout rate during the war. The sudden availability of paid employment on the home front after a decade-long Great Depression drew tens of thousands of adolescents into the civilian workforce. Addressing a fifteen-state regional child welfare conference in January 1944, Sutherland estimated that more than 1 million high school age youth had "stayed on jobs instead of returning to school last fall." Having "stopped short in their studies of civics and ethics and other humanizing influences," these "children" might find their emotional and intellectual development impaired.[36]

The Foundation's focus on youth reflected a growing national concern about unsupervised children and a spike in juvenile delinquency. During the summer of 1943, this concern peaked with hearings in the US Senate and the creation of "teen canteens," recreation centers funded by the federal Office of Community War Services. These canteens appeared in dozens of American cities, including Houston and Dallas, to provide supervised recreation for youth whose parents were occupied with the war effort.[37] One of the more widely read journalistic series about the problem ran in the *Dallas Morning News*; the Foundation packaged and distributed the series as a pamphlet titled "Preventing Wartime Delinquency."[38] In its first year in print, 10,000 copies of the pamphlet were circulated around the state; it was subsequently picked up by the National Recreation Association for nationwide distribution.[39] The pamphlet advocated for the creation of a crime prevention bureau within the Dallas Police Department to coordinate the city's various youth-serving agencies such as the juvenile court, the boys and girls clubs, parks and recreation services, visiting teachers, community centers, church groups, and child guidance clinics; a similar bureau had already been established in Houston. The pamphlet's analysis of the causes for wartime juvenile delinquency echoed the conclusions of military psychiatrists about soldiers who experienced mental illness in combat. "Dallas boys and girls are normal," it asserted, but the war setting—rather than an innate proclivity for delinquency or inherited psychoses—had engendered "an environment of loose morals and lawlessness."[40]

As the war began to wind down, mental health experts turned their focus from adjustment to wartime circumstances to "readjustment" to civilian life for both returning veterans and their families. Indeed, as early as October 1943, Sutherland was preparing for "the next great mental hygiene problem . . . re-education of the returned soldier and sailor."[41] By 1944 Sutherland was working closely with the Eighth Service Command on the development of a "rehabilitation plan" for returning veterans. As it had during the induction screening process, the Foundation served as a liaison between local communities and the bewildering (at times) array of federal agencies and programs available for returning veterans.[42] In some communities, such as Houston, the Foundation helped form local organizations to assist returning veterans in finding employment and accessing social services.[43] For instance, at the 1944 annual meeting of the Texas Social Welfare Association, the Foundation sponsored an "inter-agency luncheon" with a lecture from Thomas Saling of the US Civil Service Commission. The talk, titled "Self-Conscious Science and the Returning Veteran," sought to provide service agencies with an appropriate mental health framework for preparing employers to hire returning veterans.[44] Noting that only a small number of returning veterans would need prolonged psychiatric care, Saling warned that "the most likely way to turn a perfectly normal young fellow into a problem is to treat him like one." Families and employers were advised to strive to foster "normal" situations and interactions, while also being patient with possible "chronic fatigue," "jumpiness," and "sloppiness" from veterans. That said, Saling stressed that all concerned should view the adjustment process through a lens of normality; "GI Joe," after all, "has spent from one to three years or more on the biggest and toughest camping trip in the world" and craved nothing more than normalcy. The Foundation also completed a study of 1,000 veterans to develop trial methods for assessing and treating readjustment problems. The Foundation found that some returning veterans, particularly those who had sustained physical disabilities, grew embittered at what they perceived as a "lighthearted" attitude and "lukewarm" effort toward the war within civilian society.[45] Mental health needs, therefore, did not end with the war itself; in fact, identifying and meeting those needs was essential to the cohesion of postwar society according to a growing number of experts, policymakers, and organizations.

For his part, Sutherland drew on the wartime experience to lay out an expansive view of postwar mental health. The war had brought "emotional difficulties" out of the shadows and into the realm of the "respectable."[46] To an unprecedented extent, people "can now admit their emotions and worries, without fear of appearing 'different.'" In an increasingly "complex society," mental health education was essential for "sensitive persons" to live successfully. "This is where the educator must not fail," Sutherland warned, "and he won't if he possesses the qualities of humanity, flexibility and sensitivity."[47] In his many public speeches and writings from this period, Sutherland framed mental health in broad, comprehensive language, which called for helping individuals to "adjust" to their social environments and, at the same time, for those environments to be shaped around the physical and emotional needs of individuals. In this respect, Sutherland's (and by extension the Foundation's) advocacy for mental health reflected a public health approach. In a characteristic 1945 pamphlet, "Essentials of a Community Mental Health Program," Sutherland envisioned "community action" for mental health as encompassing not only the provision of community mental health clinics but also of functioning garbage services, roads, street lights, and other elements of social infrastructure.[48] Thus, as we shall see, many of the Foundation's early forays into community mental health projects incorporated an array of issues that, from a contemporary perspective, might seem to lay far afield from mental health but that made perfect sense from an early-twentieth-century public health perspective. In casting its net widely, the Foundation not only found a range of community needs but also found itself ensnared in social and cultural controversies.

Bringing Mental Health to the Heartland

One of the first of these controversies to involve the Foundation took place on its own doorstep. In 1944 a simmering dispute between President Rainey and the Board of Regents over academic freedom at the University of Texas resulted in Rainey's removal. Board appointees of conservative Democratic Governor Lee "Pass the Biscuits" O'Daniel attempted to abolish faculty tenure and cut funding for social science research, associating both with what they viewed as a politically subversive faculty overly sympathetic to the New Deal. The Board further alleged that Rainey presided over a "nest of homosexuals" and sought to admit African American students. According to one regent, "the teaching of social work" ought to be eliminated because "it only created socialists." When Rainey aired his grievances against the Board at a general faculty meeting in October 1944, the Regents used the occasion as a pretext to fire him on November 1. In response, university students went on strike, with 8,000 students marching in protest from the campus to the nearby capitol building and the governor's mansion. Tempers eventually cooled when a new board was appointed by Governor Coke Stevenson the next year, but Rainey, a native Texan, did not immediately fade from the scene. Instead, he spent the following year making his case publicly in speeches and radio broadcasts, culminating with an unsuccessful campaign for the governor's office in 1946.[49]

These developments created a challenging situation for the Foundation and its new director. Although he was a native Texan, Homer Rainey had been hired from outside the state to elevate the university to an elite institution "of the first class"; the hiring of one of his top mentees, Robert Sutherland, had formed a part of that endeavor. Moreover, the association with political radicalism of the academic disciplines most closely related to mental health did not augur well for the fledgling Foundation's immediate future. Already, Sutherland had compromised in accepting a nontenure track faculty appointment along with the Foundation directorship because, as an embarrassed Rainey had informed him, of Board opposition to "the principle of academic tenure."[50] Compounding the situation, Ima Hogg had lobbied furiously behind the scenes on Rainey's behalf with individual Board members as well as elected officials, while also expressing sympathy privately to Homer and Mildred Rainey, as well as Sutherland, about the "really awful" situation.[51] By the end of 1944, some wealthy Houstonians and members of the University of Texas Ex-Students Association had put forward Ima's name to Governor Coke Stevenson for a possible appointment to the Board (at the time, Ima was serving on the Houston School Board).[52] Meanwhile, Sutherland fielded attractive job offers from other universities, preparing for the event of a politically tinged dismissal. In early 1945, a concerned Ima met with several new appointees to the Board, including the newly appointed chairman and Dallas attorney Dudley K. Woodward, who assured her that both the Foundation and its director were safe from any such reprisals.[53] After tensions subsided, Sutherland would prove to be a quick study of the political landscape. Although, as we shall see, the Foundation occasionally came under fire during the Red Scare, when mental health would be associated with "un-American" activity, Sutherland carefully kept the Foundation aloof from partisan politics (see chapter 4).

Counterbalancing the political climate was the apparent hunger for information about mental health around the state. Newspaper clippings from the period suggest that a visit from a Foundation-sponsored expert was often a much-anticipated event. The *Dallas Morning News* touted the Foundation's "outstanding authorities in mental hygiene, education, and the human relations fields . . . sent on statewide tours," including Harry Overstreet, Grace Sloan Overstreet, Dr. Herbert Chamberlain, George Stevenson, Daniel Prescott, T.V. Smith, and Frank O'Brien.[54] The Foundation's public lectures often played to packed houses at churches, community centers, school auditoriums, and rotary clubs. To their surprise, speakers frequently found themselves surrounded by eager audience members after a presentation. One psychology professor at the University of Texas wrote Sutherland after a 1949 talk at the Taylor Women's Club of his "trepidation" at lecturing on "psychological concepts to a lay group." After the talk, he was "literally swamped" and "could not get away . . . many of the things they wanted to discuss afterward were either personal or about a personal problem of a friend or a relative."[55] Bernice Moore met with a similar reception to a talk given in a church in Poteet, just south of San Antonio, on women and family life. The audience was comprised "entirely" of women and young children, along with four male ministers. After the talk, discussion was muted until the women could speak with Moore privately: "When the meeting was over the women immediately gathered in a group on the church steps and one of them asked the consultant to come out there. They verbally pounced upon her—'We are bursting with things we want to talk about!—every one says—tell your children the facts of life, but no one says-what to say!' The *REAL* meeting was held with that feminine group which lasted an hour." These women, for perhaps the first time, were provided "specific information" and "referred to books" to read with their children on formerly "taboo" subjects about puberty, sex, and relationships.[56]

A fascinating portrait emerges from the notes of one of the Foundation's most-traveled paid consultants, Augusta J. Street (see Figure 2.3), who toured the state from 1948 to 1950. A trained social worker from the University of Connecticut, Street had chaired the Committee on Social Hygiene for the League of Women Voters during the 1930s. Around 1938, she relocated to Houston with her husband, Elwood, who directed the city's YMCA for several years (the couple would return to Connecticut in the 1950s). In their work, both Augusta and Elwood emphasized the prevention of juvenile delinquency: Elwood through supervised recreation and community education programs and Augusta through "visiting teachers, recreational directors, probation officers, and policewomen."[57] The couple shared an inclusive approach to child and social welfare, insisting that programs should be extended equally to racial and ethnic minorities as well as to poor and working-class whites. Augusta focused on women's issues, particularly the academic and health education afforded to young women in the public schools. Such concerns ostensibly placed Augusta on the left end of the sociopolitical spectrum in mid-twentieth-century Texas, and yet her notes reported generally favorable responses to her lectures and consultations in conservative, traditional-minded rural towns. Perhaps equally as key, her notes highlighted a general feature of the Foundation's visiting expert program. Visiting speakers often arrived in small towns bringing "modern" views and mores across a range of social and cultural practices. For many ordinary Texans, then, a first encounter with the concept of mental health became closely associated with locally controversial topics such as adolescent sexuality, early marriage, women's education and autonomy, and racial equality. In short, mental health generally equated with a brand of modernity that appealed to the desires of some rural audience members.

Billed as a "family life consultant" from the Hogg Foundation, Street visited more than two dozen communities encompassing every major region of the state. During a typical visit, she met separately with groups of male and female high school students, schoolteachers and administrators, parents and families, and local community and religious leaders. Street often found herself thrust in the middle of simmering local controversies. For instance, during her March 1949 visit to the Sabine River School District in East Texas, Street discovered that the community was sharply divided over the issue of

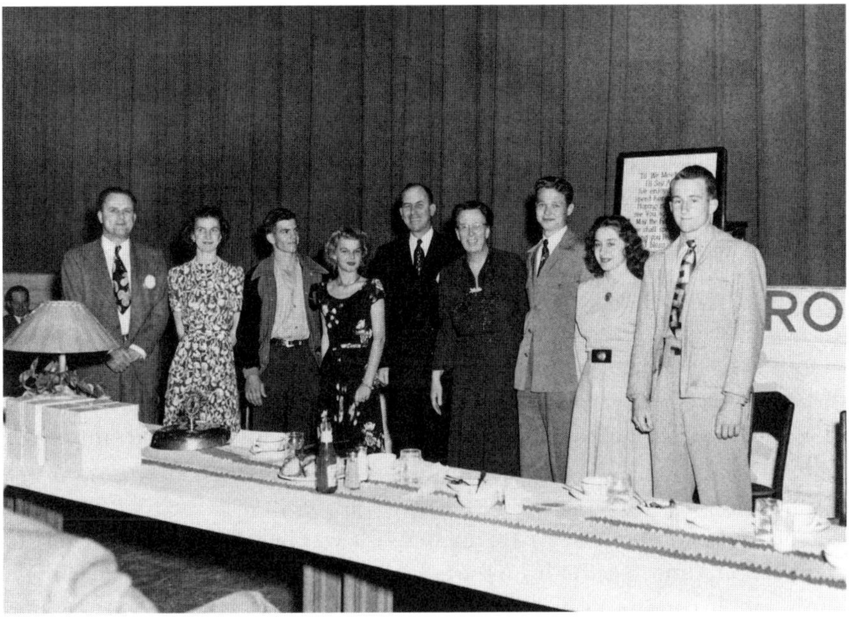

2.3. "Mrs. Elwood Street (fourth from right) at Rotary Club in Orange, Texas," undated c. 1949. Box 2AA52b, Hogg Foundation Papers. Courtesy of the Briscoe Center for American History, University of Texas at Austin.

whether to allow school dances. Students and school administrators favored school dances and parties and, as a group of boys told Street, "a chance to be together in social situations in the school." On the other side stood the school trustees, influenced by "the Church of God and some of the other denominations" in the area, who had voted against such events. Street's visit culminated with a dinner meeting with about thirty town leaders; as she recounted, "[t]hey gave me very respectful attention but I am sure that I did not get very far with them on the dancing question. . . . I was really careful not to get the administration in trouble with this group." Nevertheless, during her visit Street did meet with the youth fielding "plenty of questions on sex," followed by a meeting with mothers "with questions that brought out the fundamentalism of their religious concepts." The school superintendent and principal, she concluded, were "very fine people up against a community wall of ignorance and prejudice" that would be difficult to surmount.[58]

A similar milieu greeted Street when she arrived in Matador, a rural town of about 1,300 people in north central Texas, whose economy stemmed from the 420,000 acre Matador Ranch.[59] "A knock out for a sociological graduate student to research," Matador was in Street's telling a place characterized by little new in-migration and plenty of "inter-marriage of tenant farmers, isolation that shuts out ideas, the patriarchal family, church authority and tradition."[60] Street wrote disdainfully of the local Parent-Teacher Association, whom she portrayed as overly formal due to "pent up feelings of wanting to do like city-folk"; she described the group of seventy high school students with whom she met as "spindly" and malnourished. "They were repressed and stiff and I labored for a laugh," she recounted. "They have no dancing in the school or in the town, a movie is the only commercial entertainment, they do well in athletics, both boys and girls have teams but nothing but prayer meeting and revival meetings ever comes their way."[61] A similarly bleak landscape greeted Street when she arrived in Collegeport, an impoverished community of mostly tenant farmers of rice and cotton located near the Gulf Coast south of Galveston. Street depicted a "once thriving community" that had fallen on hard times; in fact, the town had suffered the loss of small businesses and population in the decades prior to her visit (the town's population was about 200 in 1948). The school district had only been in existence for about a decade.[62] The dinner accompanying her visit was held "after eight o'clock to give the men time to get in from the fields." Street sympathetically noted these hardscrabble conditions in her notes: "I will never forget the way the children had to wait until the adults were served and the adolescent boys last of all because of buffet style, the grown-ups wanted to be sure there would be some for the others before the young wolves got to it. They didn't mind but as soon as they got their plates full they disappeared and did not eat with the families." Confronted with such scenes of poverty, Street found herself addressing more than just her usual mental health subject material—"physical needs" as well as "emotional needs" stood front and center. "It was hard," she recalled, "because I wonder if I could know enough to imagine what the rural home and its life were like."[63] A similar situation confronted Street in Grandfalls, a community comprised largely of migrant oil field workers where family instability and poverty presented major challenges to the local schools. She described malnourished students who reacted slowly even when presented with "'sure-fire' stuff [about sex] that causes most high school groups to whoop and howl" in a group meeting. The superintendent and principal reported that students often came to school hungry, "that family morale is very low, that drinking is universal, broken homes quite usual and no recreation except as the school furnished it."[64] The school did offer softball games and square dances, but the local church regularly opposed the latter.

Church opposition surfaced during Street's visit to a larger community: Lubbock, home of Texas Tech University. After delivering a lecture on the topic of "personality development and goals for maturity" in a high school auditorium, Street was questioned by the local Baptist minister, who "waved his Bible" at her and "challenged [her] to support [her] statements by biblical reference."[65] But the minister was in the minority, as Street recounted:

> It was something new to me and I thought as fast as I could. The audience knew him as a fanatic and did their best to protect me but I made up my mind that I would give as good as I got. It was spirited but quite exhausting. He had a notebook and pen and was writing down what I said. The ladies told me that he puts out a sheet that he hands from door to door (can't put the stuff thru the mails) and would surely get out one on me. Be prepared! This would be the time that one of the Mothers had to ask me to explain how to tell a child the Father's part in reproduction![66]

Of major concern to many school officials was the growing number of married students, particularly "married girls," whom they feared would share with their classmates what they presumably had learned about sex. Nationwide, the age of first marriage dropped in the first postwar decade, with a concomitant drop in the age of first-time pregnant mothers (both hovered around seventeen to eighteen). Historians have suggested that adolescent sex was accepted within the context of marriage but produced anxiety outside of it—particularly within high schools, where attendance and graduation rates would reach historic highs by the 1950s.[67] High schools thus served as agents of socialization to an unprecedented extent; in Texas, this trend seems to have resulted in a heightened tension over sex, exacerbated by religious and social prohibitions particular to the South. As the historian Susan Cahn has framed it, Southern adolescent girls in particular "forced older generations to confront the influence of sexual modernism on a society still steeped in antebellum and Victorian traditions of racial and sexual hierarchy."[68] This confrontation was on full display during Street's visits to various Texas towns; her reports frequently tabulated the number of high school and even junior high school students who were married and the anxiety among adults about it.[69] "Everywhere I go this year," Street noted, "the school authorities talk to me about the question of early marriage."[70] They were not comforted by Street's suggestion that "without a doubt there are others in their rooms that have had sex experiences, probably having them right along, that they are talking too." Visiting Shamrock, a town in West Texas, Street discovered that "every high school had a few married girls in it." The problem was so concerning to administrators that some schools had banned married students from participation in extracurricular activities, on the premise that they had "taken on the responsibilities of an adult."[71] In her visit to Henderson, in rural northeast Texas, Street responded to these concerns by focusing on how vocational education for girls could prepare them for future roles as wives and mothers:

> To do my part on the other side of the picture, I talk about every girl having a vocation or training as making them more desirable as a wife. I ask the boys to tell me why and they finally get around to "she will know the worth

of a dollar, what it means to come home tired at the end of a day and that she can help buy the furniture, etc." I try to tell the girls that it is fun to be really grown up and support yourself, to prove yourself in an adult world, that you have been Papa's little girl but now you want to be a companion and not a burden to a husband, that you can get some pretty things and even be more attractive.[72]

In Orange, a midsize industrial town east of Beaumont, Street confronted the problem of expression rather than suppression of adolescent sexuality. "It seemed to me as I worked with the senior class," she observed, "that I had never been in a school where the boys and the girls had such maturity of a not too desirable kind. I found that there were several married students and the questions that came in showed more acceptance of intimate sex relations as a natural part of their life than I have ever had from a similar age group."[73] By contrast, Street found examples of extreme repression that led to tragic results. Street's visit to Cunningham, an unincorporated community of about 200 people located in north Texas, provided perhaps the most poignant instance. She described the "covered dish supper" held for her in the school auditorium after a choral program in her honor. "It was eight o'clock before we started to eat and with all those luscious dishes sitting on the tables in front of them, not one of the dozens of small fry around snatched a single bite of food. Self-control of that kind for children only comes with a fairly rigid family pattern." The seating arrangement expressed the "challenge" Street faced—men seated together in the center of the room, with women and children on the sides. Noting that "the Pentecostal church was the main experience in their emotional lives," Street worried about the need for "relaxing attitudes" toward social relationships. This concern arose despite the fact that the Cunningham school principal had taken the then-controversial step a few years earlier of introducing a school counseling program. A self-described "firm believer in mental hygiene," the principal admitted that he was viewed by local citizens as a "crackpot" and his "mental hygiene group meetings have been called 'a gathering of the nuts.'"[74] However, a grim reminder of the need for such programs was provided just a few weeks prior to Street's visit. A fourteen-year-old girl who arrived home late from a date with a boyfriend was beaten with a "bull whip" by her father. "She went to her room and was so quiet that [her father] became scared and as he opened the door the child shot herself." With that fresh in her audience's mind, Street hoped that "not all that I said on the subject of love and understanding our young people was lost."[75]

Many parents and teachers expressed gratitude to Street. After a February 1948 visit to Menard, a town located in the Texas Hill Country about 140 miles northwest of Austin, she reflected on the mostly positive reception to her talks: "I have had so many persons come up afterwards and comment on the fact 'I sure thought you were talking about me' or 'that was right down to earth,' 'I never knew before that all kids acted as mine do' 'it helps a lot to know that our mistakes with the children aren't very bad.' To me this time of shaking hands and accepting the remarks is like gathering in the harvest."[76] Interestingly, the scenes of both the most extreme poverty and the greatest appreciation came in African American communities. For example, Street's notes from the "colored high school" in Bay City, near Houston, described this setting:

> I wish that I could give a picture of this. A dilapidated building, a room on the second floor with every seat full (two) and then some standing. I expected the floor to go thru any minute. Such interest and courtesy and afterwards such appreciation from the students, the principal, the teachers. It is a very hard job to know what to say and how to say it and I never feel that I can evaluate what I do. I know that I sweat blood over this kind of a group. . . . I think they need all the encouragement that a white group can give.[77]

In Pearsall, a town located in the South Texas Valley, Street spoke before an auditorium filled with high school students—divided evenly between "Latin American" and "Anglo" students. By her own account, she struggled to answer "questions on boy and girl relationships that would fit the mores of both groups." She also suggested that the experiences of Mexican American students in public education formed an important and promising subject for future study.[78] But the major takeaway from Street's myriad encounters was that they were inspiring a public demand for mental health services before any providers were in place to satisfy it. The circuit rider visits showcased the need for a trained workforce, mental health education for teachers and school personnel generally, as well as individuals capable of providing mental health services at the community level. This deficit in turn reflected Texas' lack of academic and professional programs in psychology, psychiatry, counseling, and social work, which apparently exceeded national shortages in these professions. Of particular note was the lack of a single graduate school of social work in any public university in Texas. As early as the 1920s, the Texas Social Welfare Association had provided workshops and trainings for individuals who worked in positions that normally would have required formal academic training in social work. Many of the Texas Social Welfare Association's members left the state seeking formal training and often did not return. During the 1940s, attempts to establish a school of social work at the

University of Texas failed due to political opposition, initially from Regents during the Rainey affair and later from East Texas legislators who feared that improving social welfare services would "aid the spread of communism."[79]

The Hogg Foundation helped advocate for the School of Social Work and other academic programs. "It's a disgrace that we don't train our own social workers in Texas," Sutherland lamented during a dinner speech at the Ripley House in Houston. "They have to leave here to get their training, and when they're gone—they're gone."[80] The Foundation also provided workshops for practitioners of mental health and related fields such as education.[81] For instance, the Foundation joined forces with the Houston Bureau of Mental Hygiene (formerly the Child Guidance Clinic) and the University of Houston in fall 1944, offering to cohorts of Houston-area schoolteachers a series of educational psychology classes. The courses were offered for college credit by both participating universities.[82] Lecturers from as far away as Sutherland's doctoral program at the University of Chicago introduced students to the concept of personality development and detailed the signs of emotional disturbances. In a course titled Mental Health Skills of the Teacher, educators practiced responding to hypothetical "classroom situations" ranging from mild disobedience to serious violence. A theoretically oriented course, The Mental Health of Human Development, explored the four developmental stages encompassing the years of one's education: preschool, childhood, adolescence, and young adulthood. Other courses devoted to the "exceptional child," teacher, family, and returning soldier seemed to anticipate the postwar expansion of American primary and secondary schools, as well as universities.

The Houston program was one of many inaugurated by the Hogg Foundation, which increasingly articulated its mission in expansive terms. "Everywhere," wrote Sutherland in 1945, "there are basic problems of human relationship. They appear in the growing-up difficulties of children, in the quest for harmony within families, in the conflict between social and economic groups, and in the personal failure and maladjustment of some adults."[83] A "demonstration program" brought guidance counselors to El Paso's junior and senior high schools, while another project trained counselors for North Texas State College. The Foundation sponsored mental health workshops for teachers in San Antonio, Houston, Alpine, San Marcos, Kingsville, Denton, and Austin. Renowned speakers occasionally led these presentations. E. Franklin Frazier addressed black collegiate audiences in Galveston and Austin in 1946; Margaret Mead lectured on the state of the American family to the Dallas Council of Social Agencies and the Houston Family Service Bureau in 1948.[84] Building on its initial outreach during the war years, in its first decade and a half of existence, the Foundation sponsored more than two hundred lecturers and reached "well over a million people."[85]

Occasionally such endeavors forged interracial and interethnic cooperation, suggesting an inclusive model of "community mental health" that undoubtedly reflected Sutherland's racial liberalism. These programs also suggested that a broad spectrum of social services and disability categories fell within the rubric of mental health at that time. For instance, starting in 1945, the Foundation began providing financial and expert support to the program of the West Side Community House, a settlement house opened that year in Clarksville, a historically African American neighborhood in Austin. Led by neighborhood residents, the house offered marriage and parenting classes, a well-baby clinic, daycare, a preschool, an afterschool program, and job training for teenagers. Photos from its 1949–50 program emphasized "inter-racial goodwill," displaying student volunteers from the University of Texas as well as Huston and Tillotson Colleges, Hogg Foundation consultants, and day-to-day activities of various programs. Bernice Moore of the Hogg Foundation sat on the board of directors for the Community House.[86] For another program, the Foundation sent University of Texas speech therapist Jesse J. Villarreal to Houston and Beaumont numerous times between 1944 and 1954. There he led clinics for special education teachers, health officials, and parents on speech and hearing disorders.[87] His impact on largely Anglo audiences seems to have been profound. "Now I can see that there is something to this speech correction work and that it needs a trained person," admitted an impressed Houston assistant superintendent to reporters. Villarreal "opened the eyes of many," effused one parent in a letter to Sutherland.[88] These sorts of activities reached a culmination of sorts with an extended community mental health project that inserted the Foundation into historically troubled race relations in East Texas.

The Woman's Foundation Grants, 1946–48

For a two-year period starting in November 1946, the Hogg Foundation partnered with the Woman's Foundation of New York to sponsor an "intensive" project in fifteen communities around the state of Texas. This project was something of an anomaly for the Hogg Foundation's erstwhile collaborator. Founded in 1942, the Woman's Foundation's stated mission was "to engage in the study of the problems of the American Home and of the American Woman and to disseminate knowledge of tested solutions of such problems."[89] Its president, James M. Wood, who was also the president of Stephens College for Women in Missouri, elaborated on this mission in his published writings. He argued for the inclusion of women in leadership positions at the newly formed United Nations, for the creation of a college for "unwanted" (i.e., unmarried) women over the age of forty, and for the various important roles that women should play "not only in the home but in business and in public life."[90] The premise for these proposals appears to have been a viewpoint reminiscent of the "woman's movement" that had existed at the turn of the twentieth century, one that advocated for women's public roles based on their supposedly innate physiological, psychological, and intellectual differences from men. Moreover Wood appears to have joined in the chorus of messages to American women after World War II, encouraging them to return to the domestic sphere of marriage, childrearing, and homemaking.[91] Because of their "biological function" as mothers, Wood suggested, women possessed an "instinctive sympathy" that could bring a more humane influence into policymaking councils and corporate board rooms. Wood also believed the postwar era presented the most propitious time for a greater inclusion of women in important roles. "The most important event of the twentieth century thus far," he exhorted, "has been not its great wars nor its political or economic revolutions, but the emergence of women into the world of men."[92] The Woman's Foundation charter reflected Wood's formulations in language that also seemed to echo the growing emphasis on traditional roles for women in the postwar era. Placing the preservation of "the traditional American home" at its center, the charter went on to "assign to women" the "task of conserving and strengthening the essential values of home life," which held national significance: "the stability of the nation can be assured only through the stability of the home."[93]

In practice, this language seems to have taken its cues from the families of the growing middle class. A 1950 retrospective summary of the organization's work to date reported mostly on the problems of the nuclear family in a suburban setting, highlighting programs such as a training program at Vassar College for (presumably well-to-do) women over forty.[94] Moreover, the organization's board of trustees, national advisory council, and officers included only three out of a total of about fifty individuals from the states of the Deep South, with the overwhelming majority of members coming from the Northeast or California. One of those three was former University of Texas president Homer Rainey; another was Hogg Foundation director Robert Sutherland. It appears that Sutherland used his influence to persuade the Woman's Foundation to partner in supporting an ambitious series of community projects in Texas, the idea for which originated with Sutherland himself. Indeed, the project's aims reflected closely Sutherland's expansive, public health–inflected conception of community mental health. The stated goal was "to improve the standards of living" in each community, based on needs identified by community members themselves, and then provide expert assistance in addressing those needs. Small grants were subsequently awarded to communities in the areas of "health, juvenile delinquency, housing, sanitation, and many other specific projects." In February 1948, the results were reported at the National Conference on Family Life, an event called for by President Harry Truman, sponsored by the Woman's Foundation, and attended by over 125 nonprofit organizations in the nation's capital.[95]

Of the fifteen intensive community projects held in Texas, only a few appear to have yielded tangible results within the scope of the two-year grant period. One of the more compelling projects took place in the town of Slocum, an unincorporated town located about 100 miles east of Waco in Anderson County. By the early twentieth century, this town of about two hundred people was mostly African American, with several individuals who owned land and assorted small businesses.[96] In July 1910, after a series of disputes between individual whites and African Americans, a group of whites organized a mob of hundreds from around the county to carry out an armed attack against the area's black residents. According to a recent history, "white mobs marched through the area shooting blacks at will," a rampage that went on for several days at the end of July and beginning of August.[97] The official death toll of eight blacks was disputed even at the time by the county sheriff, who suggested that "dozens" of others who had disappeared might also have been killed. Many other black residents fled the area, never to return, while property that had belonged to blacks was seized by local whites. Although eleven whites were arrested and seven indicted, none were convicted. Until recently, this "Slocum Massacre" had been a relatively unknown event in Texas history; the state legislature officially acknowledged it in a 2011 resolution.[98]

This event clearly loomed over the Texas Family Life Study, which began in Slocum as the Slocum Rural Family Life Project in November 1946 under the Hogg Foundation's direct supervision. No clear rationale was provided for choosing Slocum other than a general statement that it "was selected because it is representative of a large number of Texas rural areas."[99] The project incorporated about 1,300 people living in a six-town region centered around Slocum, with the black population residing in a segregated section called Union Hope. The local leaders who coordinated the project were school superintendent Joe Hassell and his wife Dora, a home economics teacher, both of whom were white. Representing the black residents was the Reverend C.C. Harris of the Union Hope Baptist Church.[100] It is worth noting that black residents were invited to participate nine days after a white community leadership committee had been formed. Where once Slocum's black population had prospered in a mixed economy, it was mostly engaged in tenant farming or day labor in area cotton fields by the 1940s. But with the promise of outside funds and expertise, the community pulled together rapidly, as evidenced by a January 1947 meeting held at Union Hope School less than a month after the formation of an African American steering committee. Led by Reverend Harris, an itinerant minister based in Huntsville, and joined by circuit-riding Foundation experts, the scene was captured in one consultant's notes:

> There was plenty of evidence that the local steering committee had been at work. A team of mules pulling a scoop was at work on the school campus. Men at work too, and the school children were doing their bit. Lovely meals had been prepared for the visiting consultants in the school lunch room.
>
> When principal Andrew Jackson opened the meeting forty-three community people were present. The aged, the middle aged, the teenagers and one baby-in-arms were present. The community people had come because they had heard a program to improve their living conditions was in progress.
>
> The opening song, "Lord I want To Be a Christian in My Heart," was led by Rev. C.C. Harris, the pastor of Union Hope Baptist Church. He lives in Huntsville, Texas but he had heard something was going on at Union Hope School. His members had told him. Evidently they told him well, because it was not his custom to come to Union Hope except on his regular service days. After his song he led the group in prayer. What people joined in with Amens all through his prayer. . . . [when the chair of the family relations committee talked about ways to make the family more harmonious,] It was very noticeable that the audience agreed with this report. Amens, and Yes's were heard all through the report.[101]

Even amid this auspicious start, the town's history lingered in various ways. The project documents, reports, and correspondence describe these conditions and are laced with statements presuming a lowered capacity for organization, initiative, and planning among Slocum's black residents. For example, one consultant worried about "the lack of confidence of local leaders in themselves,"[102] while a homemaking consultant "commended the Negro on dependability, learning not to be satisfied with poor equipment and learning to do something for themselves."[103] Foundation consultants described black participation as steady but noted that individual black residents were quiet and withdrawn in interactions. An undated memo from spring 1947 mentioned a "race riot" that had taken place "twenty years ago" but that black participation in the community project reflected progress.[104] Finally, in May 1947, black residents began to open up to Ernest E. Neal (see Figure 2.4), an African American consultant who had worked with Sutherland on the American Youth Commission in the late 1930s as a graduate student at Fisk University; by the time of his work in Union Hope, Neal taught at all-black Huston College in Austin.[105] Black residents told Neal of a violent history little known outside of Slocum:

> The people are beginning to confide some of their community secrets with me. One of the things that the people of Slocum would like to erase from history is a racial conflict that took place forty-five years ago. No one seems to remember exactly when it occurred or what it occurred about. But it did happen, and several Negroes were lynched. The people don't like to talk about it. But a few Negroes and Whites still remember the incident and the bitter feelings that lingered long after the incident passed. Therefore, when Mr. and Mrs. Hassell met with the people of Union Hope in their church to discuss the project in family education, they did not receive the response expected. Mr. Hassell says that they were met with a sea of cold indifference and almost stony silence.[106]

Part of the reason for this reception stemmed from the conduct of Joe and Dora Hassell, who appear to have functioned as intermediaries between black Union Hope and white Slocum during the life of the project—in Ernest Neal's words, "the bridge over which the white and Negro community commuted."[107] On the one hand, they directed grant and local funds toward substantial physical renovations to the segregated Union Hope elementary school, notably the provision of sanitary drinking water and working toilets—things that some segregated black schools lacked during the Jim Crow era. They took the additional step of helping to bring the school's curriculum and academic calendar in line with the white district, raise black teachers' salaries to parity with local white teachers, and in the process gain state accreditation for the Union Hope school.[108] On the other hand, they clearly viewed local African Americans as inferiors in need of white-led uplift, which led to some contradictory actions. While promoting self-help solutions for problems caused by discriminatory policies, the Hassells seemed paradoxically unwilling to admit when self-help actually occurred. For instance, a 1947 survey of black residents revealed near-unanimous desire that high school education be made available to black youth. The rural district operated only one high school, for white students only; Joe Hassell responded that state policy required "that twenty students for each high school class was necessary before a high school could be operated. Union Hope graduated only seven from the eighth grade. If Union Hope wanted a high school, they would have to keep their boys and girls in school, rather than letting them drop out."[109]

When Robert Sutherland awarded Union Hope's three black teachers scholarships to attend summer leadership workshops, in recognition of their contributions to the Union Hope project, Dora Hassell objected that the same awards should go to Slocum's ten white teachers, even though they did not need the funds and had overcome comparatively fewer obstacles in

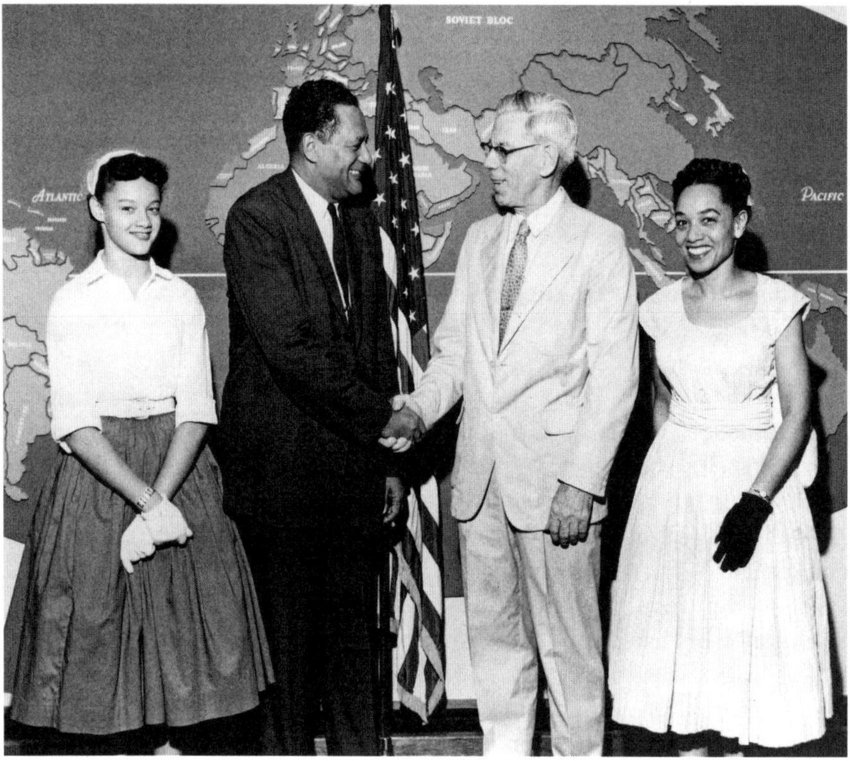

2.4. Ernest E. Neal, undated. Box 2AA52b, Hogg Foundation Papers. Courtesy of the Briscoe Center for American History, University of Texas at Austin.

improving their schools. As a surprised and indignant Ernest Neal observed, the black teachers had mounted fundraising drives to purchase much of the new equipment for Union Hope School, while the local school board had provided the same equipment out of its regular budget to the white Slocum schools.[110] Wryly noting "a very definite attitude of prejudice on the part of Mrs. Hassell," Sutherland smoothed over the situation by extending the offer to sponsor any interested white teachers who wished to participate in the summer workshop, which was focused on helping teachers become better community leaders.[111]

In spite of these incidents, the Hassells apparently had gone too far down the road of racial progress for Slocum's white leaders. In April 1948, the school board demanded their resignations, citing as reasons that they had "pushed the community too fast" and "had shown a rather high-hat attitude" toward some families.[112] As Dora Hassell explained to Sutherland, the pair had put themselves on the wrong side of white leaders at a time when other, locally well-connected individuals were "wanting the jobs we now hold."[113] Sutherland noted that this was the second instance in which a school superintendent who had been leading a Foundation-sponsored community project had been asked to resign. "While I think some inner politics were involved," he mused, "I also know that their aggressive action in community work, including the establishment of the Negro council, probably had something to do with their dismissal."[114] Nevertheless, the project's final report listed many achievements, not least of which was a more organized community in the areas of education and youth recreation. It seems possible to conclude that the project injected new life into the Union Hope community.[115]

Even as the Woman's Foundation grant came to a conclusion, Sutherland and his staff already had turned their attention to perhaps the single leading issue for proponents of community mental health: the public system of mental hospitals. Having learned key lessons from the wartime experiences with mental health and mental illness, raised the public's awareness of mental health in the broadest sense, and fired public demand for community services, the Foundation by the end of the decade would lead a full-throated campaign on behalf of individuals with mental illness. The results would transform the landscape of mental health services in Texas.

3

"A Real Revolution in Mental Health Concepts"

The Campaign for the Rights of People with Mental Illness, 1942–57

"Mental Hospitals Have No Alumni to Endow Them—Only the People," read the headline of the January 11, 1949, edition of the *Daily Texan*, the student newspaper at the University of Texas.[1] The article cited public statements by Texas Governor Beauford H. Jester; A.T. Hanretta, psychiatrist and director of Austin State Hospital; Judge Hall Logan, chairman of the Texas Board of Control; and Robert L. Sutherland, director of the Hogg Foundation for Mental Health, each calling for sweeping changes in the legal and clinical treatment of people with mental illness. These changes included improvements to the physical conditions in the state's mental hospitals, "repeal of antiquated laws" governing the commitment of people to mental hospitals, and the accreditation of those hospitals, which would require greater numbers of professionally trained staff and clinicians. "Mental hospitals have no alumni groups to wage a campaign for improvement," observed Sutherland. "The public is not attracted to problems of mental illness and mental hospitals." Sutherland therefore expressed his hope that "the facts will be reprinted by every newspaper in the state, and that all types of citizens' groups will discuss the need of improvements." Citing a 700-percent increase in the population of mental hospitals during the preceding decade, psychiatrist Hanretta warned of a "complete inundation" of already "badly overcrowded" facilities. According to Hanretta, more than a thousand persons with mental illness were "languishing in the jails of Texas because of a lack of hospital beds."[2]

The article's author was a twenty-four-year-old journalism senior named John P. Porter, whose background reflected some of the broader currents in mental health described in the previous chapter. Porter had served in the Army during World War II, where he saw action in Italy, and then worked for *Stars and Stripes*, the Army's newspaper. During that time, Porter had reported on "mental institutions in the war theatre," including hospitals for prisoners of war. He would later describe them as "essentially the same as the ones we have here—places to keep the mentally ill off the streets and away from the so-called healthy people."[3] Widely reprinted by the Hogg Foundation as well as other newspapers around Texas, Porter's article found an audience primed by years of educational lectures and pamphlets on mental health. The Foundation had stirred public demand for new mental health services and aroused greater sympathy for individuals with mental illness. As this chapter describes, the Foundation also worked behind the scenes with state officials and state hospital administrators to reform the mental hospitals. In conjunction with the Texas Society for Mental Hygiene (TSMH), the main advocacy group of its kind, the Foundation worked privately and publicly to give birth to humane improvements in the state's treatment of people with mental illness. In 1949 the legislature authorized the creation of the Board of Texas State Hospitals and Special Schools (BTSHSS), the first state agency tasked with providing more specialized administration of facilities for people with mental illness. Throughout the 1950s, the Foundation agitated successfully for a significant increase in financial resources for state institutions and programs, culminating with the passage of the state's first mental health code in 1957. This milestone would prompt then–Texas oil attorney and Democratic Party operative (and future Texas governor) John Connally to marvel at the Hogg Foundation's role in leading "a real revolution in mental health concepts" that had swept the state.[4]

These transformations stemmed partly from a national uproar about overcrowded and run-down mental hospitals and institutions. As the historian Gerald N. Grob has shown, conditions at many hospitals around the nation had declined significantly due to "nearly two decades of neglect" during the Great Depression and World War II.[5] Recognizing the problem, several state legislatures formed investigatory bodies in the 1940s. Crusading journalists helped to popularize the issue for the general public. Leading the charge was Albert Deutsch, a widely read columnist for the liberal newspaper *PM*. In 1937 Deutsch published an influential history of the treatment of people with mental illness, which was commissioned by the National Committee for Mental Hygiene (NCMH), establishing himself as "the preeminent medical journalist of the postwar era."[6] Just after the war's conclusion, Deutsch published a series of vivid articles, accompanied by shocking photographs, detailing the horrific conditions in American mental hospitals. The series culminated with the 1948 publication of Deutsch's widely read book, *The Shame of the States*, which included an introduction by the psychiatrist and proponent of community-based mental health services Karl Menninger. Calling mental illness "America's number one health problem," Deutsch noted that more than 6 percent of the population, or about 8 million people, were living with mental illness.[7] However, due to "chronic overcrowding, understaffing and lack of adequate therapeutic equipment," state hospitals had failed to provide adequate treatment. "Not a single state mental hospital in the United States" had "ever met" the minimum standards established by the American Psychiatric Association (APA) for appropriate ratios of psychiatrists, nurses, and attendants to patient populations.[8] Deutsch called for a greater emphasis on "preventive psychiatry" in community-based clinics and more support for "active therapy and research" within the state mental hospitals. This, he hoped, would result in more "ideal" state hospitals that would be less crowded, better funded, and adequately staffed. In turn, such reforms would allow for experimentation with more therapeutic treatments, the abolition of mechanical restraints and the greater use of open wards, separate and adequate facilities for senior citizens, and closer working relationships with nearby medical schools and mental health services.[9]

Other exposés appeared in high-circulation periodicals such as *Life*, *Commonweal*, and *Christian Century*, likening mental hospitals to Nazi concentration camps and insisting that they adopt reforms focused on "cure rather than incarceration." Perhaps the most dramatic of these portrayals was *The Snake Pit*, a novel published by Mary Jane Ward in 1946 and adapted into a motion picture in 1948. Ward had based the novel on her own experiences as a patient for eight months in a mental hospital in New York, where she was subjected to scalding baths and electroshock therapy. In the film, top-down shots of the overcrowded ward evoked a human snake pit. The point was hammered home further by the APA and the NCMH, each of which published reports and advocated publicly on the issue. In addition to establishing standards for all hospitals and clinics, the APA created an inspection board to assume the task of inspecting facilities for the care and treatment of people with mental illness. The collective impact of this wave of popular and professional agitation was to elevate mental health to the top rungs of the nation's political agenda. In the states, a similar discovery was taking place, including in Texas.[10]

Behind the Scenes, 1942–49

Today, the Hogg Foundation's role in mental health policy reform is known only in the most general sense, with little detail provided in the published histories of Ima Hogg, the Hogg family, and the Hogg Foundation. One of the most explicit statements can be found in the *Handbook of Texas*, the definitive encyclopedia of Texas history. "[T]he establishment of the Hogg Foundation at the University of Texas at Austin and the fortuitous appointment of Sutherland as director of the foundation in 1940," states the entry on "Mental Health," "provided a source of funds and an organizational focus for reform across the state. Sutherland's importance in influencing legislative action and mobilizing resources to restructure the state's system of mental-health care was crucial."[11] In this drama of mental health reform, Foundation director Sutherland played a central but largely hidden role, reflecting a characteristically low-key approach. Sutherland rarely sought the spotlight, either for himself or the Foundation, when it came to policy reform, even though he viewed the need for reform as urgent. Indeed, the problems with the state's system of mental hospitals had confronted Sutherland within the first year of his tenure as director of the Hogg Foundation.

Already these problems had been documented in two major surveys of Texas' mental hospitals conducted by the US Public Health Service (PHS) in 1938 and 1942. By the time of the latter survey, the state of Texas was operating seven mental hospitals under the supervision of the Texas State Board of Control (TSBC), a state agency formed in 1920 to administer state parks and buildings, serve as purchasing agent for state agencies and institutions, and oversee all the state's "eleemosynary" institutions for dependent populations. A three-member body comprised of political appointees, the TSBC thus maintained a broad array of responsibilities and exercised jurisdiction over a large number of far-flung institutions housing individuals with physical disabilities, developmental disabilities, diseases such as tuberculosis, adjudged juvenile delinquents, and dependent youths such as orphans, in addition to people with mental illness. By 1942 the TSBC included an eleemosynary division directed by Charles W. Castner, a psychiatrist who had been elevated to the position after serving as superintendent of the Wichita Falls State Hospital. Thus, while the governance structure of the state's mental hospitals included some administration by credentialed experts in mental illness, stark inadequacies remained and were identified by the PHS surveys. The study's 105 separate recommendations addressed deficiencies in physical plant, sanitation, staff–patient ratio, salary, safety, record-keeping, staff qualifications, occupational therapy, recreation, and classification. Because of the many shortcomings, asserted the study, a "repressive atmosphere" that was more custodial than therapeutic had set in.[12]

That same year, the Hogg Foundation began collaborating with the TSBC. In January 1942, TSBC chairman Weaver H. Baker wrote to Foundation director Sutherland to request assistance and to express his concerns about conditions in the facilities under his supervision:

> In as much as the State Board of Control has jurisdiction over several thousand persons suffering from mental illness, and it is our purpose to render such service as conditions will permit in the matter of providing these people with surroundings and treatment that will tend toward their recovery, I am taking this method of expressing our appreciation of the work you have done and will do in the future along the same lines. If we can render you any assistance, kindly feel free to let us know. . . You may rest assured that

> it will be the policy of this Board to cooperate with every agency available to us that will in any way inure to the benefit of the mentally ill of this state, and I want you and your associates to feel free to make suggestions to us at any time.[13]

Baker and Sutherland subsequently met over lunch on February 5, 1942, to "discuss some of our mutual problems in relation to Mental Hygiene."[14] Over the next few years, Baker consulted Sutherland to review candidates for administrative positions at the state's institutions, while Sutherland in turn invited Baker to attend Foundation-sponsored public lectures and events.[15] In March 1943, Baker chaired a panel at the annual meeting of the TSMH titled "The Governor and the Board of Control Plan the Future of Mental Hospitals."[16] This planning included a growing amount of input from the Foundation. Sutherland toured Austin State Hospital, the state's largest facility for people with mental illness, and assisted the TSBC in its unsuccessful effort to recruit Jack Ewalt, head of psychiatry at the University of Texas Medical Branch in Galveston, to lead the institution.[17] Of particular interest to Baker were educational opportunities for the professional and direct care staff. For instance, in June 1943, the Foundation provided a weekend seminar led by Russell Dicks, a minister and faculty member at Southern Methodist University who helped "pioneer the hospital chaplaincy program" during previous tours at Massachusetts General Hospital in Boston and Presbyterian Hospital in Chicago (he would later go on to serve as chaplain for Duke University Hospital after World War II).[18] At the time he led the seminar for state hospital workers, Dicks had taken charge of a national training program in counseling for military chaplains embedded with active-duty troops. As a result of this seminar, the Foundation later sponsored a demonstration study at Austin State Hospital in which two chaplains offered religious services, counseling, and a music program to patients. Later that year, the TSBC included such programming in its regular budget for its largest state hospital in Austin.[19]

In addition to seminars and studies, the Foundation provided the TSBC with published literature to distribute among hospital staff, through its "Lectures in Print" series printed by the University of Texas Press. Such interventions outlined a more humane approach to the patients in mental hospitals, as in the article "Life in Our Mental Hospitals: Its Meaning for the Individual," distributed to all staff in Texas state hospitals and special schools in June 1943.[20] The article, which originally had appeared in the NCMH journal *Mental Hygiene*, was authored by Samuel W. Hamilton, who served as mental hospital advisor in the Division of Mental Hygiene of the PHS (the agency responsible for federally run mental hospitals at that time). Hamilton had conducted and authored the 1942 survey of Texas mental hospitals on behalf of the PHS. In the article, Hamilton took readers on a step-by-step journey that began with a commitment process that existed in only two states—Mississippi and Texas. Commitment to a mental hospital was a criminal proceeding that required a jury trial to determine "lunacy" or "insanity" in order to gain placement in a hospital—sometimes with loved ones compelled to testify against an individual. Even if a hospital placement was mandated, an individual might still languish in a local jail for months until a space opened up in the state's overcrowded institutions. As a result, entrance into the hospital exposed individuals to an environment that differed little from jailhouse conditions. Indeed, Hamilton described most mental hospitals as prison-like, mass-custody institutions that provided little privacy, "ominous" and "gloomy" places where individuals with varying severities of mental illness were crowded together. The use of physical restraints was widespread, according to Hamilton, producing an environment where even patients who were not bound to tables or chairs were nevertheless "shackled to a sense of defeat, of shame, of hopelessness." Notably, Hamilton described both the commitment process and the hospital setting as violations of patients' "civil rights" and called for sweeping changes.

Even more striking perhaps than this forceful language was the manner in which the article was disseminated to the staff in Texas state hospitals and special schools. The NCMH granted the Foundation permission to reprint five thousand copies of the article so that "all employees of eleemosynary institutions in Texas" could read it. Each institution superintendent received a shipment of pamphlets accompanied by a letter from Robert Sutherland and Weaver Baker instructing them to make "good advantage" of the literature by ensuring that each employee received a copy and was told "what the article is and why we are distributing it."[21] The letter concluded with a request for a written response from each superintendent, "indicating what plans you have found best in encouraging your personnel to read and discuss such material."[22] At least one superintendent responded within days, from Terrell Hills State Hospital, detailing the distribution of the pamphlets to his department heads and their staff.[23]

In the wake of these activities, Sutherland and Baker collaborated with the TSMH in inaugurating a newsletter, titled *Texas Eleemosynary Trends: The Work of Our State Schools and Hospitals.* The first issue was published in February 1944 as an attachment to the regular TSMH newsletter (similarly titled *Texas Trends*) and thanked the Hogg Foundation for funding the enterprise.[24] This "special issue" included excerpts from the 1942 PHS survey of mental hospitals, an editorial on commitment laws written by the medical director of the PHS hospital in Fort Worth (and author of the 1938 PHS survey), and articles by hospital superintendents reporting on ongoing improvements and requesting more assistance from the legislature. One article, after declaring that no state hospital should house more than 2,000 patients, noted that five of the state's seven hospitals housed more than 2,300 each. Two hospitals, in Big Springs and Wichita Falls, admitted only white patients.[25] The final article called for "out-patient clinics" that could assist individuals transitioning out of hospitals back into the community and offer "preventive psychiatry and mental hygiene" for individuals who did not require hospitalization.[26]

The newsletter was distributed to 3,800 state employees, with an admonition from Baker that "the inculcation of correct mental hygiene attitudes and the training of our State hospital and school employees in the proper care of the State's wards can not be over-emphasized."[27] Indeed, Baker informed his superintendents that two additional issues were forthcoming that year, which "should be a source of information and inspiration" to the staff. In soliciting suggestions for article topics from staff, Baker articulated the newsletter's purpose; it "should tell of new and old methods, of solving problems in institutional administration, of scientific discoveries," and provide "a medium for exchange of ideas and information" not only among practitioners and providers of services but also the public.[28] However, the first issue of *Texas Eleemosynary Trends* would turn out to be its last, due to external political pressure. In October 1944, Baker informed Sutherland that the TSBC was withdrawing from the joint venture because some legislators privately had expressed concern that it reflected an attempt to "gain political advantage." Baker, "with extreme regret," also cited the unrest at the University of Texas surrounding President Homer Rainey as a contributing factor (see chapter 2).[29] The Foundation continued to circulate professional literature among the state hospital staff, with the TSBC's support, but the agency was no longer permitted to directly support a publication of its own.[30] In addition, the Foundation continued to provide expert-led professional development seminars and workshops for hospital staff, leading TSBC psychiatrist Castner to praise "the cooperation of the Hogg Foundation . . . to keep alive a spirit of progress, notwithstanding the handicap under which we must work."[31]

Baker's regretful tone reflected the friendship that had developed between him and Sutherland. By 1944 the pair was collaborating on textbooks and other side projects, and Baker had begun signing letters with the salutation "your friend."[32] In a particularly revealing exchange, Baker informed Sutherland that his name was being discussed among legislators and university regents as a possible successor to Rainey for the presidency of the University of Texas. Protesting that he was not an applicant, Sutherland stated that he was content in his "present niche" at the Foundation, "cooperating with others but not expressing any ambition for change myself." Baker noted that he had "already mentioned to one member of the Board of Regents your ability and that you would make a good President" but promised to relay Sutherland's lack of interest.[33]

Sutherland's response to the newsletter setback was to begin channeling more reform-minded activities through the TSMH, whose mission more explicitly included advocacy for mental health and for which Sutherland served as an officer in numerous capacities during the 1940s and 1950s. The TSMH mission statement included "[t]he promotion of facilities for the prevention, diagnosis, treatment, and care of individuals whose behavior or personality difficulties lie within the field of mental hygiene," as well as "the encouragement of any necessary legislation to achievement of these ends." It also called for "the inclusion of the principles of mental hygiene in the professional preparation of doctors, teachers, social workers, nurses, and other professional groups."[34] For his part, Baker joined the TSMH as a dues-paying member in 1945. The TSMH continued to publish *Texas Trends* independently, and Sutherland continued to circulate it among TSBC members and institutional staff at mental hospitals, even after Baker's sudden death in a car accident in September 1946.[35] In a subsequent letter to Hall Logan, the new TSBC chairman, Sutherland attached an article, published in the January 1947 issue of *Texas Trends*, on the state's mental hospitals. The author, psychiatrist Jack Ewalt, was a faculty member at the University of Texas Medical Branch in Galveston and recently had taken over the directorship of the Galveston State Hospital and the presidency of TSMH. The article set forth the issues confronting mental health reformers heading into the spring 1947 legislative session.

Ewalt began by recounting the numerous unimplemented recommendations from the 1942 PHS survey, particularly the establishment of an "inspection system of the state hospitals by qualified psychiatrists," the adoption of APA standards for the mental hospitals, and the abolition of the use of the criminal justice system for commitment procedures as well as county jails for holding patients awaiting acceptance at a state hospital.[36] He also noted acidly that the hospitals "have fewer trained psychiatrists now than at the time of the [1942] report" and lacked full-time psychologists on staff. The TSBC had yet to establish a "social service program," a "Division of Statistics," "Out-Patient Clinics . . . in centers of population throughout the state" or distinct services for children with mental illness. The "repressive attitude in certain wards" decried in the 1942 survey still existed, with "most" or "perhaps all of them" employing "some type of physical restraint such as camisoles, cuffs, and other types of apparatus which no well-equipped and well operated psychopathic hospital should own." Ewalt ranked Texas' mental hospitals in the "middle third" of quality with other states in the South and Southwest regions. However, he qualified this observation by pointing out that the comparison was with "other hospitals that are already notoriously inadequate." Any evaluation of Texas by "modern medical standards" or by comparison with the "much better" hospital systems of the Northeast or Midwest "would be absurd." The main culprit for these continued inadequacies was the lack of funding; Ewalt contrasted the cost of $8 per day to care for "the average general hospital patient" with the average expense in Texas per patient, which fell below $8 per week. In conclusion, Ewalt threw down the gauntlet for his readers:

> The first tendency of the public is to blame first the Board of Control, and second the superintendent managing these institutions. As a matter of fact, the Board of Control has done the best that they could possibly do under very difficult circumstances. The superintendents and staffs who are operating these state hospitals should have some type of recognition because they have carried on in the face of disappointment, frustration, inadequate personnel, and inadequate understanding from the patients, the patients' families, and the public. Only their fierce devotion to duty and the belief that someone must care for [people with mental illness] has kept many of them on the job. . . . The superintendents of the various hospitals have year after year carried their requests to the State Board of Control [which] has offered their recommendations to the Legislature who in turn, listening to the appeals for economy from their local constituents, have had to cut the appropriations asked for by the Board of Control. . . . *The responsibility for this state of affairs lies not with the doctors, not with the Board of Control and not with the Legislature, but with you, the public, who have not been sufficiently interested in the care of [people with mental illness] in the State of Texas.* (emphasis in original)[37]

Echoing previous analyses, Ewalt's long list of recommendations was divided into three broad categories: adequate staff and care for patients, more flexible and humane commitment procedures, and qualified administration of the hospitals. In Ewalt's view, the TSBC, which lacked the needed expertise, could not fairly be expected to carry out these reforms. Instead, he called for the creation of a "supervisory board" that would function much like a state university board of regents. This board could be comprised of a mix of expert and lay appointees, which in turn could hire "a full-time director" of the state hospitals with "training and experience both in administrative and clinical work in psychiatry." He warned that none of these proposals would bear fruit, however, without "arous[ing] the public's interest." Ewalt anticipated "a great deal of political opposition," some of it due to honest disagreements but much of it stemming from a desire to preserve "the political control that now exists in the state hospital system." He warned that "the variation of political fortunes" had corroded the hospitals' ability to foster a therapeutic environment. In his letter accompanying Ewalt's call to arms, Sutherland admonished TSBC chair Logan that "we need your leadership.

We would like to support progressive measures, which no doubt you are planning to institute directly or to bring to the attention of the Legislature."[38]

Logan, however, turned out to be a less enthusiastic partner than his predecessor. In response to Sutherland's plea, he stated that he did not agree with all of Ewalt's recommendations for the state's mental hospitals, although he did not provide details. Logan supported increasing the pay for hospital staff and "research and training" for "doctors and nurses."[39] He appears to have been skeptical of broad-based reforms in hospital programming, such as greater educational and treatment programs for patients, or expanded community-based clinical services. While he did not comment on Ewalt's proposal for a separate board to administer the state's system of mental hospitals, Logan may have held obvious reservations; as Ewalt himself had suggested, such a move would greatly diminish the TSBC's scope of authority. Thus, in the 1947 legislative session, Logan focused instead on the most obvious shortcomings: poor physical conditions, overcrowded wards, and low wages and salaries for existing staff classifications.

The Texas legislature seemingly adopted Logan's viewpoint during its spring 1947 session, when a special committee was formed to investigate conditions in all the eleemosynary institutions supervised by TSBC. The committee's final report, issued in April 1947, focused entirely on physical conditions: "unsanitary" wards at Rusk State Hospital, building shortages at Terrell Hills State Hospital, and "utter confusion" and a "dire need of new buildings" at Abilene State Hospital.[40] The longest section of the report described "overcrowded wards" at Austin State Hospital, particularly in the segregated wards for African American patients. When patients exited the rotted floors and peeling walls in their wards for a meal, they were greeted by "unsanitary and foul odors," inadequate plumbing, and open piles of garbage. At Austin State School, the committee found a dormitory for "the lower type of patients" that was "far too crowded, with many of the patients totally unclothed." Moreover, these patients slept on "very badly soiled, torn, and worn out" beds to such an extent that some were reduced to "sleeping upon bare springs."[41] Conditions at San Antonio State Hospital included vermin infestation:

> The main kitchen is so filthy that food prepared there should not be fit for human consumption. Utensils had film of dirt . . . galvanized wash tubs were being used to place prepared food in. The main dining room was dirty. Many English sparrows were flying around inside the dining room, often lighting on tables while patients were eating. Bird droppings covered some tables where patients eat, and while they were eating. This condition should not be tolerated under any circumstances. . . . The store-room in the main kitchen [had] filthy floors, sacks of corn meal that had been cut by rats and

> meal scattered. Dried apples, etc, open with no cover and had rat dropping in same. Food improperly kept open all over the place. . . . Patients are not being fed the same food as employees.[42]

The report concluded that conditions at the state's institutions fell "far below the standards . . . of a civilized nation" and "should be remedied immediately" through investments in physical plants and staff salaries.[43] In response, the legislature passed a $25 million appropriations bill that allocated more funds for physical plant improvements and staff salaries; however, the final bill removed nearly all of the $3 million that had been intended to finance new building construction. Subsequently, Governor Beauford Jester used a line-item veto to strike a provision that would have provided for the construction of a new dormitory building at Austin State Hospital for African American patients.[44] Moreover, even increased top-line staff salaries appear to have lagged well behind national norms. For instance, the superintendent at Austin State Hospital was slated to earn an annual salary of $5,450—about half of what Ewalt had suggested as the national norm. The clinical director's salary was set at $4,200, below the range of $5,400 to $7,500 that Sutherland had recommended to the TSBC and more commensurate with the suggested range for a "Junior Psychiatrist."[45] Sutherland maintained regular communication with Logan during the legislative process, strategizing and sharing information. The TSMH mounted a letter-writing campaign aimed at key legislators, while Sutherland and Ewalt provided expert advice for Logan's use in discussions with legislative committee members. At the end of May, Logan phoned Sutherland to share the news that much of the sought-after funding had survived; however, Sutherland and fellow reformers would view this result as incremental progress only. With so much left to do, mental health reformers would heed Ewalt's advice and take their case to the public during the next biennial legislative session scheduled for spring 1949.[46]

"The Shame of Texas," 1949–50

The reform campaign became more public with the appearance of John Porter's article in the *Daily Texan* in January 1949. Porter had begun studying state mental hospitals six months earlier, with financial support from the Hogg Foundation and director Sutherland connecting him to state officials, superintendents, and various reformers. Having gained the public's attention with his initial reportage, Porter began work on a more detailed, eight-part investigative series that he hoped would "attract the attention we need to convince the Legislature" to support wide-ranging reforms.[47] Although the Foundation did award Porter some funding for his research, Sutherland was very careful to distinguish that his personal support for Porter's work came

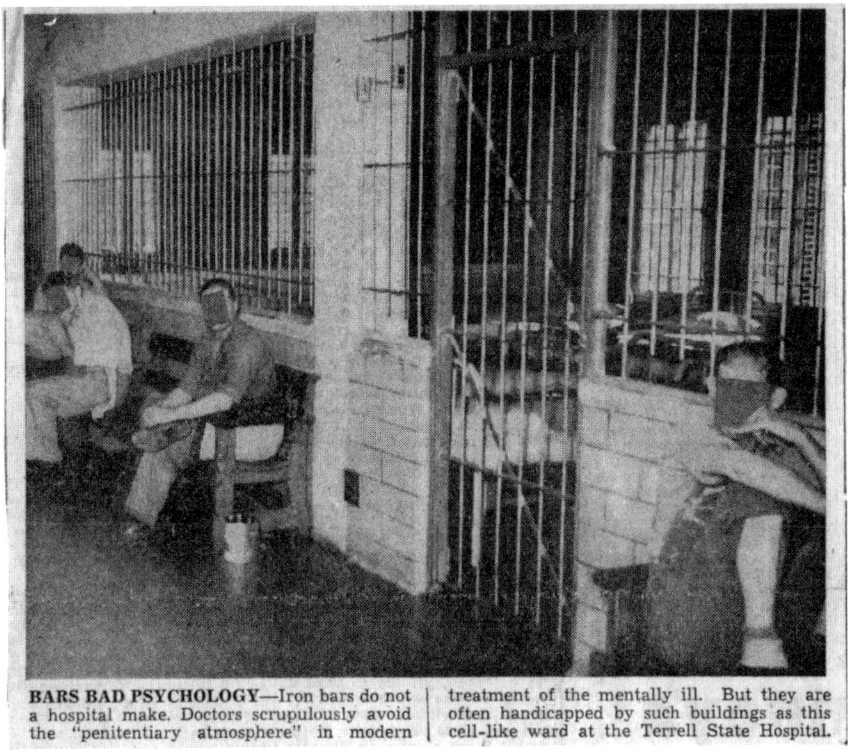
BARS BAD PSYCHOLOGY—Iron bars do not a hospital make. Doctors scrupulously avoid the "penitentiary atmosphere" in modern treatment of the mentally ill. But they are often handicapped by such buildings as this cell-like ward at the Terrell State Hospital.

3.1. Photograph of a "cell-like ward" at Terrell State Hospital. *Austin Statesman*, March 22, 1949. Box MAI9-U111–112, Hogg Foundation Papers. Courtesy of the Briscoe Center for American History, University of Texas at Austin.

in his role as an official of TSMH and not as director of the Foundation. On February 14, the pair signed an agreement stating that while Porter was conducting "research for the Hogg Foundation concerning the conditions of . . . various state mental hospitals in Texas," his publications in "newspapers and periodicals were not in any way connected to the Hogg Foundation."[48] On March 20, fifteen newspapers in Texas simultaneously began publication of Porter's eight-part series, whose title, "The Shame of Texas," clearly drew inspiration from Albert Deutsch (some newspapers titled it "Texas Tragedy"). Each installment in the series focused on one institution, telling the story of "the nation's worst" mental hospitals from the viewpoint of the "doctors and officials . . . who are handcuffed to antiquity in an age of modern science." As one psychiatrist told Porter, "Texas' six mental hospitals have degenerated into six penitentiaries."[49] Like Deutsch, Porter included vivid photographs illustrating overcrowded, dilapidated conditions and some of the outdated treatment methods still in use in Texas hospitals (see Figure

3.1). At Big Spring State Hospital, "patients are crowded into teeming cages, the attendants are guards, and the superintendents are wardens;" meanwhile, photos from Rusk State Hospital showed patients sleeping in rows of mattresses on the floor due to lack of beds, while beds were squeezed into the bathrooms at Abilene State Hospital.[50] The last article in the series described a patient who was allegedly beaten to death by two attendants at Wichita Falls State Hospital during the previous year and an attendant at the Austin State Hospital who had "shot and killed his wife and a patient who happened to be in the line of fire, and then slashed his own throat."[51]

Proponents of mental health reform pressed their case in other forums. In February 1949, Sutherland dispatched Porter to speak at a symposium held in Houston by the Texas Social Welfare Association, with the entire Harris County legislative delegation in attendance. He urged officials to support the TSBC's appropriations request for $61 million—more than double its previous biennial budget—to allow for sweeping physical plant renovations and staffing improvements. By one account, Porter's talk held his audience riveted: "you could have heard a pin drop" while he described the "crisis in our outmoded institutions."[52] In the meantime, Sutherland, Ewalt, and other reformers were meeting privately with TSBC chairman Logan and other state officials. Proposed legislation included the doubled budget request, the creation of a separate board to oversee the state mental hospitals, the commission of a feasibility study of "the development of out-patient clinics and other preventive measures," and a constitutional amendment that would remove the requirement of a criminal jury trial for commitment procedures.[53] Later that month, the TSMH amplified these reforms at its annual meeting in Dallas, with the theme of "Care for the Mentally Ill." The keynote speaker, psychiatrist William Menninger of the Menninger Foundation of Topeka, addressed a standing-room-only audience of 2,200.[54] On March 15, Logan, Sutherland, and other reformers attended a House committee hearing on the proposed measures. The results of these efforts were mixed. Although the legislature approved the increased appropriation for the state hospitals, Governor Jester once again vetoed the bill for lack of funding. However, House Bill 1, approved in June, created the nine-member BTSHSS. The enabling legislation declared "the responsibility of modern society to afford adequate treatment for its less fortunate citizens who suffer from the impediment of mental and physical ailments" and acknowledged the "growing sentiment in Texas that its system of State Hospitals and Special Schools has not kept pace with modern thinking, training methods and procedures." It further stated that the TSBC was too broadly construed to provide "the specialized supervision required." In an unusual move, the routine bill-reading procedure was suspended to allow the law to go into effect immediately, reflecting the perceived urgency of the situation.[55] The proposed constitutional amendment removing the jury trial was approved by the legislature and went to the voters along with ten other proposed amendments in a special election in November 1949. Governor Allan Shivers, who had taken office that summer, publicly campaigned on behalf of the measure, while Sutherland and Bernice Milburn Moore appeared on radio broadcasts promoting it. However, the amendment went down to defeat, in no small part because it appeared on the ballot alongside politically controversial proposals to abolish the poll tax and to allow women to serve on juries, as well as even less popular measures such as a proposal to increase legislators' salaries.[56]

Mental health reformers responded to these setbacks by redoubling their efforts in both the private and public spheres. Sutherland began collecting information from the superintendents of the state hospitals about physical plant, staff, and patient populations.[57] Meanwhile, the newly formed BTSHSS invited several Texas news reporters to tour the state hospitals and special schools. As a result, newspapers continued to publish scathing exposés throughout late 1949 and early 1950. Significantly, feature articles with titles such as "Mental Hospitals Badly Understaffed" or "Mental Institutions Over-Crowded, Staffs Overworked, Newsmen Find," began to appear not only in big-city dailies but in rural newspapers, suggesting that the issue was spreading more broadly around the state.[58] A single reporter for the Associated Press, who had toured the hospitals, wrote the majority of the articles.[59] Civic groups also promoted the issue; in addition to TSMH and the Texas Social Welfare Association, the Mental Health Committee of the Junior Chamber of Commerce (known sometimes as the Texas Jaycees) circulated a mass mailing titled "Mental Hygiene" that urged action on the "deplorable conditions" in the state mental hospitals and called for "a coordinated mental health plan for the state of Texas."[60] Meanwhile, the sudden death of Governor Jester on July 11, 1949, presented reformers with a more supportive ally in his successor, Allan Shivers, who as lieutenant governor had helped pass the funding measures in the legislature that Jester had vetoed. Shivers also had publicly supported the proposed amendment to end jury trials for mental hospital placements. However, Shivers inherited a financial crisis; the legislature had concluded its regular biennial session without funding the regular operating budgets of any of the eleemosynary institutions for the second year of the biennium due to a budget shortfall. His predecessor Jester, unwilling to support deficit spending and seeing no sources for new revenues, had vetoed the budget requests for insufficient funds. The crisis also coincided with an election year, in a state with a conservative electorate. Thus mental health reformers hoping for dramatic increases in spending for new facilities, professional salaries, and community-based programs faced a challenging political environment, in spite of the ascent of a friendly governor.[61]

Evidence of a crisis in the state's mental hospitals continued to mount, thanks in part to the newly formed BTSHSS, which (with Shivers' blessing) invited outside organizations to carry out studies and publicize results.[62] In January 1950, the PHS declared mental illness to be "the nation's number one public health problem" while simultaneously announcing that Texas' mental hospitals ranked the worst in the nation.[63] In a presentation to the BTSHSS, the study's authors showed that Texas spent one of the lowest per-patient amounts nationally. Around this same time, the National Institute of Mental Health also conducted a study ranking Texas thirty-seventh in per-patient spending on mental illness and at or near the bottom nationally in such categories as expenditures per overall population and number of trained psychiatric nurses.[64] Finally, at Sutherland's invitation, the APA medical director met with the BTSHSS to deliver recommendations. He advised that Texas could create "a mental hospital program capable of discharging 75 percent of those admitted to asylums within two months" through a variety of measures, including the expansion of community mental health clinics, the discharge of senior citizens ("the merely old do not belong in mental institutions"), and other improvements.[65] Civic organizations also joined the campaign, led by the Texas Jaycees, which circulated a pamphlet that asked its members "How Would You Like to Spend a Month—or Longer—in the County Jail for the 'Crime' of Having Appendicitis?"[66] The pamphlet likened this scenario to the continuing use of county jails to hold people with mental illness awaiting placement in the state's still-overcrowded mental hospitals. Attached to the mailer was a letter from BTSHSS, "urging" and "authorizing" the "young men of the Junior Chamber of Commerce" to visit any mental hospital, view the conditions for themselves, and communicate their concerns to elected officials. The letter encouraged group "caravans" to tour the facilities, photograph them, and then share the information with others. Attached to the letter were muckraking news clippings of investigative reports on the hospitals. "We cannot afford to assume that reform is inevitable," admonished the letter; "COMPLACENCY AND APATHY WILL NOT GET THE JOB DONE!"

Amid this hue and cry, in January 1950, Shivers called for a special legislative session whose main purpose was to allocate funds for the state's eleemosynary institutions.[67] The public campaign continued prior to and during the session, with Shivers himself authoring an editorial that was published widely in Texas newspapers explaining his proposal to raise funds through an increased oil and gas tax.[68] The Texas Jaycees released a thirty-minute documentary film, titled "Shock Treatment," filmed with the express permission of state authorities.[69] Images of each of the most notorious facilities played across the screen while the narration lambasted the "penitentiary atmosphere" and likened the patients to "sardines . . . packed in very close quarters." The film concluded by calling for "early treatment" clinics in the communities and an increase in the numbers of trained professionals. "Not

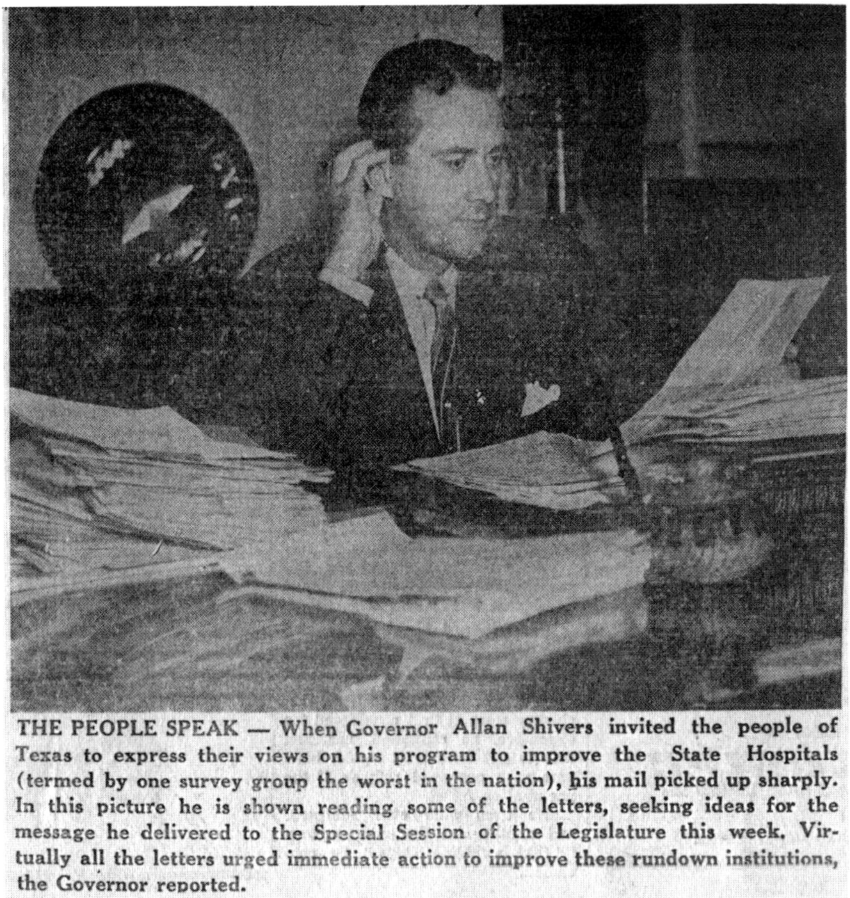
THE PEOPLE SPEAK — When Governor Allan Shivers invited the people of Texas to express their views on his program to improve the State Hospitals (termed by one survey group the worst in the nation), his mail picked up sharply. In this picture he is shown reading some of the letters, seeking ideas for the message he delivered to the Special Session of the Legislature this week. Virtually all the letters urged immediate action to improve these rundown institutions, the Governor reported.

3.2. Photograph of Texas Governor Allan Shivers reading letters from citizens on a radio program in response to his request for public suggestions for improvements to the state hospitals. *The Panhandle Herald*, February 3, 1950. Box MAI9-U27, Hogg Foundation Papers. Courtesy of the Briscoe Center for American History, University of Texas at Austin.

until an adequate program of prevention as well as hospitalization" was implemented could people with mental illness "hope for the dawn of a better day."[70] The campaign was effective; a statewide poll conducted in January 1950 showed that 60 percent of Texans were aware of the issue and, among that group, 96 percent agreed that improvements were needed.[71] When Shivers solicited suggestions from the public, he was "showered" with letters from all over the state, reflecting the heightened public interest in the mental hospitals (see Figure 3.2).[72] Shivers' request was echoed in solicitations from mental health advocacy groups, such as the TSMH mailing that urged "key persons in Texas" to write letters under the heading "Governor Shivers Has Asked to Hear From You!"[73]

Shivers further rallied public opinion ahead of the special session by authorizing the creation of the Citizens Committee on Mental Health (CCMH) in January 1950. Comprising roughly one hundred individuals, the CCMH was a who's who of mental health advocates, experts, and professionals in Texas. The committee met on January 30, 1950, at the Driskill Hotel in downtown Austin, joined by Shivers and several "key legislators," to underscore the urgency of the issues that had prompted the special session and to outline the committee's purpose. The keynote speaker was Daniel Blain, medical director of the APA whose visit to Texas was funded by the Hogg Foundation. Over the subsequent two weeks, Blain met with legislators to explain the national significance of the reform measures under consideration. In his CCMH address, Blain emphasized the need for "educating the general public regarding the real meaning of mental health, for only enlightened and understanding citizens will continue to support the State's efforts to provide adequate care for its mentally ill."[74] He also called for expanded in-service training of mental health personnel and "making jobs attractive" by improving staff housing and salaries; only then could the state increase the number of attendants in the hospital wards.[75] The Hogg Foundation circulated Blain's message via a brochure titled "Seven Challenges," attached to a mass mailing that pointedly asked CCMH members, "How many dozens or hundreds of copies can you distribute in your community?"[76] In a private letter, Shivers later thanked Sutherland and the Foundation for rallying support for the special session and pledged his future cooperation in mental health reforms.[77]

On February 1, 1950, Shivers opened the special session with a powerful speech. "No one," he declared, should be "in the dark" about the reason for the session.[78] "An emergency exists," caused by a hospital system in which "24,000 people [were] crowded into a space that properly should house 14,000." At nearby Austin State Hospital, ten doctors and four registered nurses were serving 3,200 patients. "[M]ore space, more doctors, more nurses" and "modern treatment" were essential to allow people with mental illness "to get well and to return to society." Shivers described inspection visits to the state hospitals that he had conducted during the previous months:

> I have seen, with my own eyes, mattresses spread side by side on hall floors and beds set up on open porches in winter-time, so that patients might have some place to sleep. I have seen 26 beds jammed into a ward room built for 15. I have seen epileptics eating in bathrooms for lack of dining space. I saw 77 aged and mentally ill women locked up in a condemned building. I saw 400 mentally defective children and 800 seniles housed in prisoner of

> war shacks made mostly of plywood and tar paper. . . . I saw dilapidated, non-fireproof buildings without fire escapes. . . . I could go on. The picture varies from place to place, but everywhere there is evidence that we are now reaping the bitter fruits of a long era of neglect.[79]

Mental illness, he cautioned, was "no respecter of persons" and could occur in "your neighbor's family" or "your own family, or mine." Were that to occur, he warned, "you could not, under present conditions, expect treatment leading to a cure." Shivers urged "immediate and sympathetic consideration" for his proposal to increase taxes on oil and gas, in addition to a host of other items, to raise funds for the operating budgets of state hospitals and special schools, as well as new building construction and new professional staff positions. Shivers concluded with dramatic illustrations of the state's national rankings: "Texas, the proud Lone Star State—first in oil—forty-eighth in mental hospitals. First in raising goats—last in caring for its state wards."[80]

This "Hospitals First" plan, as Shivers dubbed it, was met with "a hearty round of applause" from legislators and received favorable media coverage.[81] The first weeks of the special session "gave full and almost exclusive attention" to mental illness and mental health issues.[82] The Hogg Foundation arranged for individual legislators to visit "outstanding state hospitals in other states" with "a well-conceived program" for children with mental illness and other special needs.[83] Despite some opposition from anti-tax representatives, oil and gas executives quickly lined up in support of the measure, with the caveat that the tax increase would be temporary. A little over a week after Shivers introduced his proposal, it passed both houses by large margins.[84] At the urging of TSMH, thousands of supporters of mental health reform mounted a letter-writing campaign aimed at key legislators. At least one state senator reported having "received many letters" that helped swing his vote.[85] By August 1950, change was underway, with "several doctors, 70 years of age and older," being "retired" by BTSHSS and numerous construction projects in progress.[86] However, as we shall see, problems continued to persist in the areas of commitment procedures and the lack of community-based mental health services.

Putting Brains Before Bricks, 1951–57

In the year after the 1950 special session, the BTSHSS came under political attack. During the spring 1951 legislative session, Senator Dorsey B. Hardeman of San Angelo introduced Senate Bill 278, which proposed abolishing the BTSHSS. Citing "economy and efficiency in state government," Hardeman called for replacing the non-salaried, nine-member BTSHSS with a paid, three-member board appointed by the governor. At a March 1951 committee hearing, a parade of board members, psychiatrists, physicians, and advocates for people with mental illness and tuberculosis (many of whom had been active in promoting recent reforms) spoke against the bill and in favor of the BTSHSS. They presented statistics showing improvements made in the board's short existence to the numbers of doctors and nurses, the new and remodeled buildings under construction, and the patients receiving better treatment.[87] In addition, they argued that the board had not been given sufficient time to prove its worth, a contention widely echoed in the state's newspapers.[88] "More progress has been made in the last year under the new board than in twenty-five years before," declared the president of the Texas Tuberculosis Association.[89] For his part, Senator Hardeman presented no witnesses and no evidence to support his proposal. Defenders of the BTSHSS, however, argued that "politics" were behind it, led by James Mahon, chairman of the Jaycees' mental health committee and co-chairman of TSMH, who warned that "politics have no place" in the treatment of people with mental illness.[90] Indeed, as early as August 1950, the board had begun to experience legislative interference. In a memo to Hogg Foundation director Sutherland, the board cited cases where individual legislators had attempted to intervene improperly on behalf of patients, hospital staff members, and contractors who had complained to them. One unnamed legislator, outraged that a well-connected patient was not immediately admitted to a state hospital outside of established procedures, "made overt threats about what he would do in the Legislature."[91] Similar suggestions arose in response to S.B. 278, with board vice-chairman H.B. Zachary of San Antonio testifying about politically connected contractors who had become irate when long-standing contracts were terminated due to "below standard" materials.[92] Once again, reformers mounted telephone and letter-writing campaigns. "NOT ONE TANGIBLE REASON . . . NOT ONE SHRED OF TESTIMONY" was given for the proposal, screamed a mailer from James Mahon to the Texas Jaycees membership.[93] "The critics are seeking excuses for doing what they have already decided to do, rather than facts upon which to base judicious action."[94] Similarly, the CCMH wondered "what emergency has arisen that makes it necessary to discard, without adequate discussion, a plan that we accepted less than two years ago?"[95]

Although the bill was ultimately defeated, the brouhaha surrounding it brought unexpected "blowback" upon the Hogg Foundation, which had operated largely behind the scenes and had taken little direct role. The Jaycees' James Mahon, perhaps the most fiery of the BTSHSS's defenders, had done some work on the Foundation's payroll the previous year, and this in turn had raised questions from elected officials and the University of Texas administration about the Foundation's role in public policy debates. Similar inquiries were put to Hamilton Ford, a psychiatrist who served on the faculty at the University of Texas Medical Branch in Galveston. Ford was an active member of the TSMH and had testified before the Senate committee regarding Senate Bill 278.[96] A few months after the bill's defeat, in July 1951, the Foundation held a luncheon conference on the subject. In attendance were state legislators, assistants to Governor Shivers, the heads of several state agencies (including the BTSHSS), reporters, and administrators from the University of Texas. Participants agreed that it was "appropriate for the Foundation to work with other state organizations including public agencies."[97] However, they also concluded that the Foundation "should not become identified with any one program" and "should avoid propaganda and also partisan support of a person or agency." In particular, "lobbying" was to be avoided, although it was expected that the Foundation could play a leading role in "keeping the needs, the problems and the alternative courses of action prominently before all groups which could act" and maintaining "a vigorous, yet impartial support of high standards in mental health work." In addition, the Foundation could continue to partner with public agencies "to make grants for surveys, experimental projects, and other special types of work which cannot always be included in [their] regular budgets." This conference clarified the Foundation's scope of activity in public policy as one encompassing policy analysis, nonpartisan advocacy, and expert assistance to state and local agencies. By the end of the decade, this work had become so routine for the Foundation that Ima Hogg mentioned it only in passing in a 1961 recorded interview.[98] The 1951 legislative battle and subsequent conference had the effect of clearing a path for the Hogg Foundation to continue its public policy work, which meant finishing the task that had been partially achieved up to that point: modernizing the state's system of hospitals, establishing community-based clinics, and revising the mental health code.

An immediate signal of the Foundation's surer footing in the public policy arena was the publication of "Behind the Walls of Texas State Hospitals," a twelve-part series of reports that appeared in Texas newspapers between November 1952 and February 1953. The author, Bert Kruger Smith, had joined the Foundation as a full-time staff member that same year, after earning bachelor's and master's degrees in journalism, the latter from the University of Texas. Over the next thirty years, Smith would serve as the principal author of dozens of Foundation publications, write six books and two documentary film scripts, and host "The Human Condition," a weekly radio broadcast that ran for a decade. A native of Wichita Falls, Texas, Smith served as a circuit rider along with Sutherland, research director Wayne Holtzman (see chapter 4), and associate Bernice Milburn Moore (see chapter 2).[99] Like many of her colleagues, Smith's interest in mental health stemmed from personal tragedy; in 1949 she lost a six-year-old son to polio and spent much of her subsequent career focusing on the mental health of children and fami-

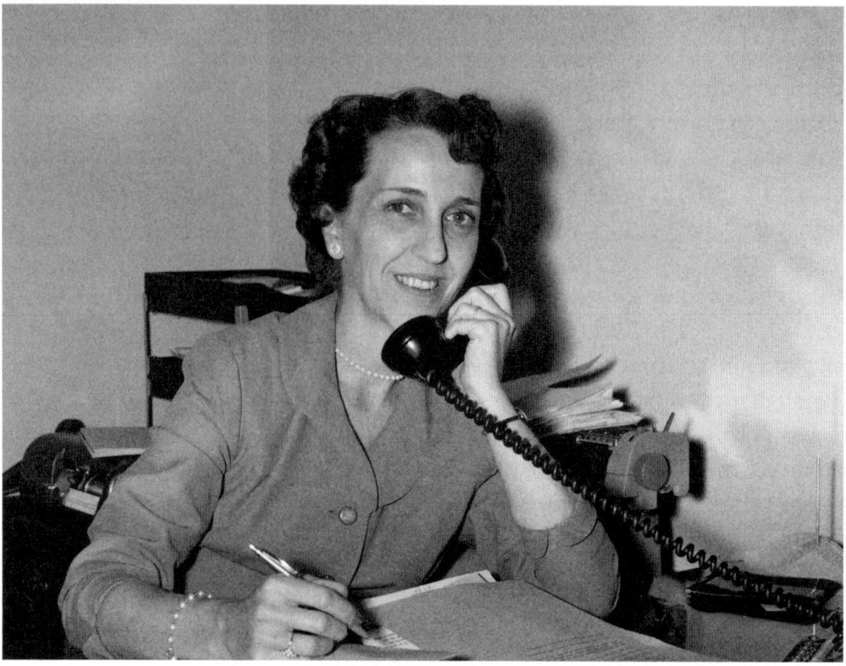

3.3. Bert Kruger Smith in her office, c. 1960. Box 3A210, Bert Kruger Smith Papers, Briscoe Center for American History, University of Texas at Austin.

lies.[100] As early as 1960, Smith's achievements were such that she was nominated for membership in the National Association of Science Writers, with one referee enthusing that "her prestige in Texas is enormous. It is her work . . . that has made the Hogg Foundation known as Mr. Mental Health in Texas."[101] Smith would play a key role in keeping the problems of the mental hospitals in the public eye during the 1950s.

Remembered as "sweet and gentle" in person, Smith reserved her strongest language for her written expositions on mental health, as illustrated in the hospital series of 1952–53.[102] Each installment vividly described the experiences of individuals working or living in the state hospitals, from their own point of view: the "pretty young social worker" whose enthusiasm for mental health was dampened by an overwhelming case load, "young" and "exhausted" attendants and nurse trainees, the "failure case" of a patient who had lived in Austin State Hospital for twenty years because he had not been diagnosed or treated properly, two friends optimistically preparing for release thanks to the successful use of occupational therapy, and psychologists wistfully looking to the "wonderful outpatient clinics" in other states and wondering when Texas would support them.[103] Taken together, the articles highlighted progress made under a fourteen-point program put forward by the BTSHSS in 1951 while also illustrating the substantial work remaining to be done. The board had instituted new personnel requirements and had enrolled more than two hundred staff members in nurse technician programs at local junior colleges while also establishing residency programs for psychiatrists and clinical psychologists. A sweeping overhaul of the hospitals' classification and intake systems was underway, with numerous patients being moved to more appropriate facilities tailored to their needs rather than to their geographic location (as had been the case previously). The introduction of occupational and recreational therapy sought to replace the extensive use of seclusion and restraint; the latter measures now required "a doctor's prescription," implying that such measures should be rare and used only as last resorts. Financial shortfalls limited other reforms, such as building construction and renovation, the hiring of additional credentialed professionals, and the development of community-based clinics.[104]

Behind the scenes, mental health reformers were growing impatient with the slow pace of action from the BTSHSS and the legislature. They looked to national and regional trends that seemed to support their feeling that Texas continued to lag behind, despite recent reforms. In 1949 the Governor's Conference, an annual meeting of state governors, directed its Council on State Governments to produce a study of the treatment of people with mental illness. Between 1949 and 1955, the Council published two influential surveys of state programs, while the Governor's Conference devoted its entire 1954 meeting to mental health. Out of these activities emerged a ten-point program that closely resembled the fourteen-point program put forward by the BTSHSS in 1952; in addition, the BTSHSS took its organization cues from the Governor's Conference's initial survey of state mental health programs published in 1949.[105] Notably, the 1955 conference called for reducing the population in state hospitals by increasing prevention services in the community.[106] Similar messages were put before Texas legislators by the TSMH in the early 1950s with little success.[107] Finally, in March 1953, Sutherland convinced the CCMH to organize "about twenty" of its more prominent members to attend the May meeting of the BTSHSS and to schedule meetings with legislators and the governor's staff members.[108]

"As a private citizen who was very much interested in the program at the Board," Sutherland proposed a "liaison committee" to serve as a go-between the BTSHSS and mental health reform groups.[109] At its July meeting, the board agreed to this suggestion from "Dr. R.L. Sutherland, Director of the Hogg Foundation" and named Sutherland as chair.[110] Around this same time, psychiatrist James A. Bethea assumed the role of executive director of the BTSHSS, putting a mental health professional in a leading role for the first time at the agency (by statute, only three of the board's nine members could be "medical professionals"). In February 1954, Bethea led a delegation of board members in attending the aforementioned Governor's Conference on Mental Health. This conference refocused the board's attention on slowing the population growth in state mental hospitals and developing community-based prevention resources; it also crystallized the advisory committee's role in raising public awareness and building support for legislation.[111] To that end, Sutherland arranged for a showcase meeting to be held at Austin State School on April 13, 1954.[112] In attendance were members of both the advisory committee and the BTSHSS, as well as representatives from dozens of civic organizations and reporters. Noting that the state of Texas spent about $2 per day on each hospital patient, Bethea set a goal of raising that to $3 a day to promote "much better care and a faster recovery."[113] The group toured the facility and then heard first-person testimonials from patients, their parents, and recently released patients. The meeting concluded with a clarion call for a "state-wide campaign" to increase funding for the hospitals and community-based prevention and transitional services and for a modernized commitment law.[114] The subsequent campaign included publicized tours of state hospitals and media reports of shortcomings that resembled those of earlier years but that now, emulating Bert Kruger Smith's reportage, tended to emphasize the possibilities for improvement.[115] Within a year, the advisory committee had conducted "inspections" of all six mental hospitals under the BTSHSS's supervision.[116]

Meanwhile, in the months leading up to the next legislative session, Sutherland and his committee members met privately with legislators and their staff members to make their case for budgetary and policy changes. In June 1954, the committee met with Governor Shivers, pointing out that the national average in per-day spending on patients was $8, well above the $3 requested by the BTSHSS. Shivers told the group that they should ask for more and expressed his belief that the legislature would support increased appropriations if the case were made effectively.[117] On August 2, 1954, the board met in the reception room of the Texas House of Representatives, with several elected officials in attendance; there, advisory committee member Edgar Ezell, president of the Texas Neuropsychiatric Association, read aloud a resolution calling for a budget appropriation that would reach the $3-per-patient daily benchmark.[118] The following month, Sutherland split the advisory committee into two subcommittees, tasked with conducting inspections of state facilities and with mounting a public campaign for increased appropriations.[119]

However, the public relations effort became mired in disagreement over use of a professional firm rather than a cadre of volunteers, with Sutherland withdrawing from a leadership role in the public relations subcommittee.[120] Thus the spring 1955 campaign was led by the public relations firm of Syers,

Pickle, and Winn, with the politically connected J.J. Pickle personally lobbying individual legislators during the session. The campaign included a public address at the headquarters of the Texas Medical Association in Austin, with speeches by Shivers and Sutherland that were rebroadcast on twenty-seven television stations around the state. The BTSHSS public information committee later reported that the campaign had included fifteen thousand mass mailings, forty-seven press releases, and twenty-five radio spots in favor of legislation.[121] The results, however, were mixed. A new constitutional amendment passed allowing waiver of a criminal jury trial for commitment to a mental hospital that finally would win approval from the electorate in November 1956. The Mentally Retarded Persons Act empowered the BTSHSS to provide separately for individuals with developmental disabilities, who previously had been lumped in (both figuratively and physically) with people with mental illness.[122] Finally, the legislature approved a $7 million increase in the BTSHSS's budget that appeared impressive but, according to Sutherland, did not keep pace with the rising hospital population. Equally as concerning, the administration of the state hospitals remained in the hands of nonexperts, and decisions too often were being made on the basis of bottom-line rather than treatment concerns. "Probably the best achievement is the growing interest on the part of the legislators in this problem," wrote Sutherland in a letter to William Menninger after the session. "The lesson we have learned is that the next time all of the citizens' efforts should center directly in the legislature, and, of course, now is the time to begin that. I am looking forward to much more substantial achievement next time."[123]

The conclusion of the 1955 legislative session brought to the surface other tensions between Sutherland's advisory committee and the BTSHSS. The key fault line seems to have fallen between the nonexpert political appointees to the board and the mental health experts and advocates who advised them; the two groups frequently disagreed about priorities, best practices, and tactics for approaching the legislature for resources. More fundamentally, they disagreed about custodial versus treatment-oriented approaches to mental illness. For example, in 1955 Sutherland delegated the annual hospital inspections to the Texas Neuropsychiatric Association.[124] One year later, Sutherland noted that the board pointedly refused to consult the experts for policy advice arising from the results of these inspections. When Sutherland's fellow philanthropy head Mary Butt (see chapter 4) was appointed to the BTSHSS in 1956, he found himself quelling her outrage at the board's seemingly dismissive attitude toward psychiatric and psychological expertise. Sutherland suggested to Butt that she persuade her fellow board members to consult the advisory committee for personnel decisions, building and policy priorities, and treatment pilot projects. The Foundation had offered to fund such a project through a grant, but the board had rejected the suggestion.[125] Around that same time, the BTSHSS produced a brochure outlining the needs for the state hospitals that aimed at "shoring up the existing system without major changes," according to an independent analysis commissioned by the Hogg Foundation.[126] Even more indicative of the disconnect was the state's inability to recruit and retain talented psychiatrists to lead their mental hospitals, not only due to noncompetitive salaries but also an unwillingness to grant full administrative authority to such experts. Indeed, these conditions had led three nationally respected psychiatrists to leave administrative positions at state hospitals since 1950. As National Institute of Mental Health head Robert Felix told Sutherland in a 1956 conference call: "Now when this thing happens to three different people and they leave the state and go somewhere else and do a first-rate job that they did not do here, there's only one conclusion that an intelligent person who is trying to be objective can come to and this is what people have come to. The fault lies not so much in the man as in the system which tries to break the man . . . people see Texas as 'murder' because of the inhospitable treatment of psychiatric heads."[127]

The Foundation presented its own vision for mental health services in April 1956 with the release of *In a Strange Land*. The thirty-minute documentary film was written by Bert Kruger Smith and produced by the Foundation with support from the film department at the University of Texas and the Texas Jaycees.[128] Shot entirely at Terrell State Hospital, the film dramatically portrayed the life of people with mental illness, both inside and outside the state's mental hospitals. Made with the cooperation of the BTSHSS, the film highlighted improvements but lamented the crowding of fourteen thousand patients into six hospitals that could only accommodate nine thousand. Images of new buildings under construction and renovated open-bay wards illustrated progress made since the tax revenue measure enacted six years earlier. However, even in these ostensibly improved spaces, overcrowding remained a problem, with beds jammed together against one another and abutting miniscule recreational areas. A lack of individual privacy accorded to patients formed one of the more constant features of the hospitals. Amid these scenes, the narration highlighted the "constantly changing" social thought about mental illness. "Once, an 'insane asylum' was a human warehouse holding the ill in restraint and adding fright to the already terrifying world of mental illness," noted the narrator over imagery of a staff name badge labeled "Rehabilitation Technician." As the scene shifted to a dance, the hopeful commentary continued: "Today, your Texas mental hospitals aim to return the patient to his home, his loved ones, his community, as quickly as possible, and to bring family, community, laughter, and possibility into the hospital scene." Achieving this goal, however, required a greater investment in doctors, nurses, and other staff positions, which the film posited would allow 70 percent of new patients to be released within six months and 80 percent within a year. The film devoted about one-third of its running time to a discussion of the advent of new psychotropic drugs, in greater use in other states, as holding the potential to augment psychotherapeutic treatments and further speed the release of new patients. It bluntly illustrated group, recreational, and occupational therapies in limited use due to a lack of space and a lack of competitive salary levels for trained professionals. "Self-expression and self-reliance are important ingredients to recovery" but were only available to a small number of hospital patients due to lack of personnel and space. Of particular importance was the transition back into home and community, where "full recovery" took place. The film seemingly concluded with a female patient dancing out of the hospital to a waiting car, with upbeat music playing in the background, and into her coffee klatch where she was welcomed back by her friends. However, in a final dramatic turn, the film shifted back to compelling images shown earlier: an elderly patient's hands holding a plate of food, a silhouetted march of patients walking across a bridge, a close-up of patients' feet shuffling across a ward hallway. With tense music playing over such images, the narrator reminded viewers of "those left behind" in the hospitals, for whom there were "not enough hands" to provide the treatments needed to allow them to escape "the strange land" of mental illness.

The film's presentations of mental health and mental illness were artifacts of an optimistic but flawed vision that was characteristic of the postwar mental health movement. The language of "full recovery," so prevalent in the film, reflected the predominant thinking of the postwar era, which focused on treatable forms of mental illness at the expense of chronic and serious conditions that required long-term care. Thus while the film purported to call for improvements to the hospital, it also implied that the hospital was not an appropriate setting for full recovery. Moreover, the film's depiction of a woman who returns home from the hospital omitted any mention of treatment services in the community, reinforcing a notion of full recovery reminiscent of the "cures" offered by nineteenth-century proponents of the asylum. Amid images of a happy return to 1950s suburbia, the film called upon viewers to extend "the hand of friendship" to patients who had been cut off from "normal" everyday life and trapped in the "strange land" of the hospital (and illness itself). They could demonstrate that friendship even further, the narrator suggested, by contacting their legislators to demand more funding for hospitals.

Momentum was growing for a more sweeping policy overhaul. At the BTSHSS's request, in 1955, the Texas Research League had produced a series of reports on the board's policies and procedures and made recommendations regarding admissions, classification, treatment, and administration. At the top of the list were the abolition of jury trials for commitments and the development of a state mental health code.[129] Thus, one month prior to the release of *In a Strange Land*, the BTSHSS formally requested that the Hogg Foundation take the lead in the drafting of the state's first mental health code. The request presented the Foundation with an unusual opportunity to address several long-standing concerns about mental health policies and practices. Within weeks, the Foundation awarded a grant for the Texas Mental Health Code Drafting Project to the University of Texas Law School. The project committee was chaired by law professor Millard Ruud, working under the close supervision of Page Keeton, dean of the School of Law. The principal authors were law school graduates Jack F. Cook and Emilie Heinatz, the latter of whom was serving as executive secretary for the Texas Social Welfare Association. Serving in an editorial capacity were Sutherland and Bert Kruger Smith of the Hogg Foundation.[130] In February 1956, a two-day publicity event was held that included the committee members, Sutherland, as well as prominent Texas attorney, state Democratic Party strategist, and future Governor John Connally. Enthused about the "tremendous currents from the Hogg Foundation" that supported his own efforts to enact "a real revolution in mental health concepts," Connally threw his unqualified support behind the proposed code.[131]

The Foundation took additional steps to build legislative support for the mental health code. Toward the conclusion of the disappointing legislative session of spring 1955, Sutherland had begun exploring the possibility of having psychiatrist William Menninger, perhaps the nation's best-known advocate for mental health reform, address a joint session of the legislature. Sutherland and Ima Hogg both communicated with individual legislators about a possible Menninger speech.[132] In 1955 Menninger had delivered a similar address as the keynote speaker to the annual meeting of the Texas Conference of Foundations and Trust Funds and had been serving as an external advisor to the Hogg Foundation and sometime correspondent to Sutherland (see chapter 4). Menninger's talk was scheduled for February 12, 1957; with the Foundation covering his travel expenses and speaking fees, Menninger carefully avoided any specific mention of pending legislation or other overtly "political" topics. Titled "Brains Before Bricks," Menninger's talk consisted of an urgent plea to focus on "buying brains" before "buying bricks" in legislative appropriations, or, by extension, to emphasize treatment over custody. "[T]he most neglected health field in our nation," mental health utilized 700,000 hospital beds annually—more than half of all beds in the United States. A large percentage of those beds, Menninger contended, were wasted on patients who could benefit from more effective therapies in hospitals as well as preventive treatments in community-based clinics. Turning to the Texas scene, Menninger asked legislators to "assume that hospitals are [places] where people go to get well and not to die," decrying the continued overcrowding in "ancient" buildings. Especially "unforgiveable" was the mixing of patients of different ages and conditions; children, he observed, were too often housed in congregate dormitories with adult patients and even the elderly. The state hospitals had "almost no" full-time trained psychologists, few medical doctors with appropriate training in psychiatry, and only two of its thirty-five "social workers" with graduate degrees in psychiatric social work. Compounding these problems were haphazard commitment procedures required by Texas alone among all states (by this time Mississippi had revised its procedures). "The greater majority of mentally ill patients can get well if we give them a chance," he admonished, but doing so would require a higher level of spending on salaries, research, training centers, and "outpatient" mental health clinics. Such measures held out the promise of reducing the patient population in hospitals by preventing unnecessary admissions and providing more effective treatment to those who were admitted. In short, "a new era of hope" had arrived, presenting the Texas legislature with a unique opportunity.[133] The legislature gave Menninger a standing ovation at the conclusion of his talk, and newspapers across the state editorialized in favor of his proposals.[134]

The result of these efforts was enactment of the landmark Texas Mental Health Code (House Bill 6) and the Commitment of the Criminally Insane (House Bill 906) in May 1957. The code began with a statement of purpose that expressed well the goals for which the Hogg Foundation and its cohort of mental health reformers had been working for over a decade:

> It is the purpose of this Code to provide humane care and treatment for the mentally ill and to facilitate their hospitalization, enabling them to obtain needed care, treatment, and rehabilitation with the least possible trouble, expense, and embarrassment to themselves and their families and to eliminate so far as possible the traumatic effect on the patient's mental health of public trial and criminal-like procedures, and at the same time to protect the rights and liberty of every one. In providing care and treatment for the mentally ill, the State acts to . . . restore [the person with mental illness] to a useful life and place in society. It is also the legislative purpose that Texas contribute its share to the nationwide effort through care, treatment, and research to reduce the prevalence of mental illness.[135]

The code eradicated the jury trial system except in special cases of involuntary commitment and even there set a requirement for "competent medical or psychiatric testimony." It set forth the state's first procedures for voluntary, temporary, protective, and indefinite admission to a state mental hospital. However, the bill's scope went well beyond commitment procedures, addressing every facet of the patient's experience with the state's system of mental hospitals. Without exception, all patients were to receive "adequate medical and psychiatric care and treatment in accordance with the highest standards accepted in medical practice." The use of physical restraint was prohibited unless "prescribed by a physician" and then "should be removed as soon as possible" and a record made of its use and the reasons for it. Transfer, furlough, and discharge procedures were set forth for various categories of patients, notably with patient and family input required for most of them. The bill set forth patients' rights to visitation, religious freedom, communication, confidentiality of their clinical records, and a right to release. These provisions also applied to privately run mental hospitals, which for the first time were required to apply for a license to operate. Both private and public hospitals were to be run by psychiatrists certified by the APA.[136]

Hailed as "a jewel of a law" in the Texas press, the mental health code represented a watershed moment, borne of years of efforts to mandate fair and humane treatment of people with mental illness.[137] A key component of this campaign called for individuals with mental illness to be viewed *as individuals* and for the disaggregation of distinctive conditions that previously had been lumped together. Importantly, the language of "rights" slowly began to creep into the discourse surrounding mental health and illness, with some advocates openly claiming humane treatment as a civil right. At the start of this period, individuals with developmental disabilities were housed with people with mental illness; children shared spaces with the elderly; mild, moderate, and severe conditions went undifferentiated and often untreated amid overcrowded and dangerously unsanitary facilities whose main focus was custody. Such facilities constituted the state's main response to mental illness, exacerbated by the distant administration of political appointees who lacked any medical or psychiatric expertise, and the management of untrained staff. Reforming long-neglected facilities and outdated policies had become one of the central causes for the Hogg Foundation. The enactment of the landmark mental health code in 1957 was achieved through incremental progress that often seemed frustratingly slow to reformers.

As we shall see in chapter 5, the code did not solve all problems and brought with it unintended consequences necessitating further reforms in the 1960s. But the reform campaign also reflected an important period of network-building for the Foundation in the areas of mental health philanthropy and research, without which the mental health code would not have been possible. By 1957 the Foundation had become the most important organization in the field of mental health in Texas and its surrounding regions. This status was achieved not only through the Foundation's role in the campaign to reform the state's mental hospitals but also through its establishment of a professional network of mental health philanthropy and research, to which we now turn.

4

Branching Out

The Professionalization of Mental Health Research and Philanthropy

A mental health mascot of sorts began to appear on the scene in Louisiana and Texas during the spring of 1947. "Pierre the Pelican" was the symbol of a major public education campaign aimed at young couples who were expecting their first child. Supported by the Hogg Foundation and the Woman's Foundation, this campaign was conceived and carried out by Loyd Rowland, director of the Louisiana Society for Mental Health and former chair of the psychology department at Baylor University. It represented a local and regional response to the national demographic increase in marriage and childbirth—known more colloquially as the "baby boom"—that began during World War II and continued into the early 1960s. Accompanying the baby boom was an explosion of childrearing advice literature for young couples, led by Benjamin Spock's best-selling book, *Baby and Child Care* (1946).[1] Although it did not reference Spock by name, the Pierre the Pelican campaign echoed many of his popular prescriptions for successful childrearing. In a series of twelve carefully conceived pamphlets mailed each month to new parents, the campaign addressed "things like parental harmony, sleep habits, kindness, food habits, thumb sucking, peacefulness, security, fears, toilet training, dressing, enjoying the baby, and friends for the baby."[2] Calling for fathers to play a more active role in childrearing, the literature encouraged parents to redirect children's misbehavior rather than engage in physical discipline. "Babies must be protected from fear and made to feel secure," encouraged one mailer.[3]

Psychologist Rowland created this campaign as an early intervention to "combat mental illness" in lower- and middle-class populations, much of which he argued stemmed from traumatizing parental discipline experienced in early childhood.[4] He noted that many couples had only recently joined the middle class due to the rapid expansion of the postwar American economy and needed expert advice to shed the mores of their parents' generation. In Rowland's view, these young, first-time parents represented "a strategic group upon which educators in mental health may center their effort" by dispensing baby and child care advice.[5] Rowland argued that these parents were deeply dissatisfied with their family traditions but could revert back to those same traditions in the absence of alternative methods. Struggling with feelings of "acute helplessness" and uncertainty, these first-time parents "will never again be as willing to learn about child development as during the infancy of their first child."[6] Rowland's assumptions about family childrearing traditions reflected those of Spock and other postwar experts.[7] In response, Rowland designed advice literature that was friendly, accessible, and written at a reading level that was free of jargon or any overt references to doctors or mental health professionals. In fact, in its grant award letter to Rowland, the Woman's Foundation specifically advised him to address the material to "a negro mother with a sixth grade education (that may be somewhat high)."[8] Indeed, the advice in each printed pamphlet was given not by a sober-faced clinician but by a smiling cartoon character, Pierre the Pelican, who represented the Louisiana state bird and the local French Creole culture of southern Louisiana (see Figure 4.1).

An evaluation of the series showed positive results. Rowland led a group of students from the Tulane University School of Social Work in interviewing 594 families, two-thirds of whom had received the Pierre the Pelican pamphlets through their gynecologists.[9] Among the households that received the pamphlets, three-quarters of all women and about half of all men read them. Even more noteworthy, families that read the pamphlets exhibited different childrearing behaviors from those who did not. Fathers were "more cooperative in the care of a baby," and parents generally reported being less inclined to employ corporal punishment for children's misbehavior. These parents were more likely to allow children independent exploration and less likely to overreact to "problem" behaviors. With a "more permissive" approach, this group of parents had adopted "a better notion of sex education" and of mental and emotional development more broadly. Rowland viewed this as a success, and he was hardly alone. Other state health departments adopted the Pierre the Pelican materials for their own parent education campaigns in the late 1940s, utilizing a bound volume of the pamphlets provided by Rowland and the Hogg Foundation that included laudatory endorsements from the American Medical Association, Karl Menninger of the Topeka Foundation, Robert Felix of the National Institute of Mental Health, and George Stevenson of the National Center for Mental Health.[10] In February 1948, the *New York Times Magazine* featured Pierre the Pelican in its popular weekly column on children's and family issues, praising the literature's "disarming way of taking parents into a partnership" and warning that "you have to think ahead in matters of mental health."[11]

The Pierre the Pelican campaign underscored a number of key interre-

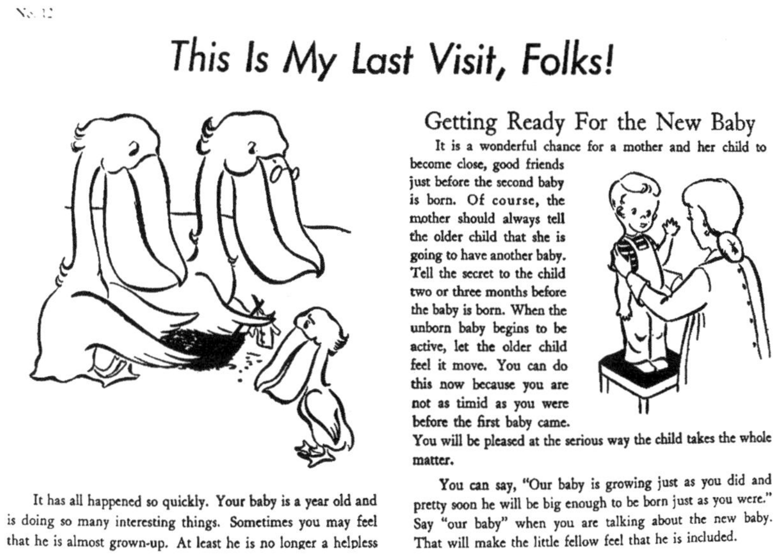
No. 12

This Is My Last Visit, Folks!

Getting Ready For the New Baby

It is a wonderful chance for a mother and her child to become close, good friends just before the second baby is born. Of course, the mother should always tell the older child that she is going to have another baby. Tell the secret to the child two or three months before the baby is born. When the unborn baby begins to be active, let the older child feel it move. You can do this now because you are not as timid as you were before the first baby came. You will be pleased at the serious way the child takes the whole matter.

You can say, "Our baby is growing just as you did and pretty soon he will be big enough to be born just as you were." Say "our baby" when you are talking about the new baby. That will make the little fellow feel that he is included.

It has all happened so quickly. Your baby is a year old and is doing so many interesting things. Sometimes you may feel that he is almost grown-up. At least he is no longer a helpless

4.1. Pierre the Pelican pamphlet no. 12. Box MAI9-U21, Hogg Foundation Papers. Courtesy of the Briscoe Center for American History at the University of Texas at Austin.

lated changes in the Hogg Foundation's approach to mental health. First, the Foundation had begun to introduce an evaluation research component into its mental health programming. Even public education projects such as Pierre the Pelican now became more targeted and were expected to be research based in their conception and to produce meaningful results that could be evaluated. In this way, the Foundation began to engage in "applied" scholarly and professional research that remained consistent with and supported its founding mission of improving mental health for all Texans. Second, the Foundation had begun to widen its scope of activity from local, community-based projects to those that might have statewide, regional, or even national impact; in fact, as we shall see, some projects crossed national borders as well. Last, the ability to incorporate research on a broader scale required an expansion of the Foundation's resources. The Foundation's resources grew dramatically during the 1950s and 1960s in a number of ways, including through the tripling of the Foundation's endowment and operating budget, a strategic approach to grant-making that attracted more research grants to Texas from national philanthropies and federal agencies, and the creation of an umbrella organization for regional philanthropies, the Conference of Southwest Foundations. These changes meant that the Foundation slowly scaled back its general outreach programming in mental health in favor of more focused, research-oriented initiatives, such as a research monograph series published by the University of Texas between 1952 and 1976 and a grant-making program that provided seed funds to mental health demonstration projects. Through its leadership of the Conference of Southwest Foundations, as well as the formation of a National Advisory Council (NAC) comprised of leading figures in psychiatry, psychology, and mental health, the Hogg Foundation further influenced changes in mental health policy and practice.

Building a Regional Grants Network: The Conference of Southwest Foundations

The somewhat apocryphal tale of the Conference of Southwest Foundations' origins has been told by several historians and is part of the organization's official history.[12] In the fall of 1948, a chance conversation at the University of Texas between the heads of three relatively new Texas foundations—Robert Sutherland of the Hogg Foundation for Mental Health, Mary Elizabeth Butt of the H.E. Butt Foundation, and Margaret Scarborough of the Lemuel Scarborough Foundation—provided the spark. Over lunch, the trio discussed their philanthropic interests and discovered that each had awarded funds to the same postgraduate programs at the University of Texas. The conversation raised questions about the lack of coordination among philanthropies in Texas and how little each of the three really knew about the charitable activities taking place beyond their own immediate experiences. In fact, as the historian of Texas philanthropy Mary L. Kelley has noted, Texas led the nation in the formation of new foundations between 1920 and 1950, due in large part to its booming population and economy. Not yet aware of this trend, the three foundation heads left the meeting with an agreement to establish an annual conference and invite other statewide foundations, with the goal of improving coordination and information sharing between philanthropic organizations.[13]

The first of what became regular annual meetings was held in April 1949 at the Driskill Hotel in downtown Austin, with an invitation list consisting "only of the foundations about which the hosts knew or had heard."[14] The meeting was billed as the Conference of Texas Foundations and Trust Funds, reflecting a statewide focus. In all, ten foundation representatives attended from within Texas, along with consultants from the Carnegie Corporation, the Rockefeller Foundation, and the Southern Education Foundation. The one-day conference proved to be "a historic occasion" where members exchanged notes on their respective experiences, missions, and challenges.[15] At the conclusion, attendees voted to hold another meeting the following year in Houston, where it would be hosted by local philanthropists including Ima Hogg herself. At these informal meetings, panels were organized around topics of interest to local and regional foundations, such as financial management or social issues that could be addressed through charitable means. The conference evolved in this informal fashion, growing from a one- to a two-day event, rotating each year to a city where a local foundation head would serve as host. Finally, at the fifth meeting in 1953, a proposal for a more formal organization, to be renamed the Conference of Southwest Foundations, was approved by the membership. The name change reflected a decision to invite members from the states adjoining Texas, and the organization's scope grew to include New Mexico, Oklahoma, Arkansas, and Louisiana.[16]

By the time of the 1955 meeting, hosted by the Texas Research League in Dallas, the organization's membership had more than tripled to thirty-five. Featured speakers included University of Texas president Logan Wilson, who spoke on "Foundation Grants as Venture Capital," and psychiatrist and head of the Topeka Foundation, William C. Menninger, who delivered a talk that he would subsequently give to the Texas legislature in the campaign to establish a mental health code (see chapter 3). Workshop sessions focused on grant-making opportunities in the physical and biological sciences, education, and community health. One panel that became a regular feature at annual meetings provided testimonials from individuals who had started their own charitable foundations; Ima Hogg and Margaret Scarborough spoke at this panel. Another panel, led by a vice president from the First National Bank of Commerce, provided guidance to prospective philanthropists on how to start a new foundation; this also became a staple of annual meetings, ensuring the growth of regional philanthropy and the organization's membership.[17]

As the conference grew, it broadened its geographic and thematic scope significantly. In 1959 the annual meeting was held in Santa Fe, New Mexico, around the theme of "The Space Age."[18] The 1963 meeting, held in Dallas, was focused around historic preservation and the role of private foundations in supporting archival and museum collections; speakers included Gordon Gray, chairman of National Trust for Historic Preservation in Washington, DC, and Harry Ransom, chancellor of the University of Texas.[19] Other meetings took place in Albuquerque, New Mexico, and Ardmore, Oklahoma, reflecting the increase in members from regions outside of Texas.[20] The growing influence of social movements can be seen in the annual meeting programs of the late 1960s and 1970s. For instance, the 1968 meeting in San Antonio, which focused on the impact of public television programming on children's education, was the first program to feature imagery of African American and Mexican American youth—as well as artwork from local elementary schoolchildren.[21] Similarly, "Let There Be Hope" was the theme of the 1971 meeting held in Kerrville, Texas, with panel topics that included "Combatting Drug

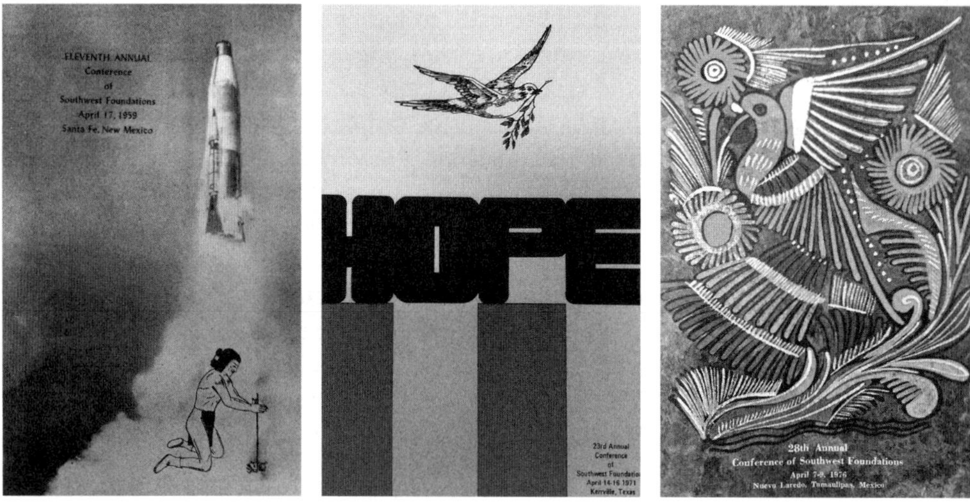

4.2. Annual Program Covers, Conference of Southwest Foundations, 1963, 1971, 1976. Box MAI9-U21, Briscoe Center for American History.

Abuse" and "Improving Minority Group Relations."[22] Twice during the 1970s, in 1976 and 1978, the conference held its annual meeting in Mexico, where it featured speakers from both countries and focused on "inter-American cooperation" to address the "problems of the borderland."[23]

The Hogg Foundation for Mental Health played a "central role" in the conference's growth during these decades. Under Sutherland's direction and with Ima Hogg's full support, the Hogg Foundation provided the conference with its primary financial base, office, and staff. Sutherland was elected several times to serve as the organization's president and vice president. Easily the foundation head with the broadest connections to national philanthropies and federal grant-making agencies, Sutherland had managed to convince the Carnegie Corporation to add the Hogg Foundation to its widely consulted national directory of foundations in 1948. His energy and personable leadership style served the new organization well as it grew rapidly in the 1950s and 1960s.[24] In Sutherland's view, the missions of the two organizations complemented one another perfectly. By the time of the conference's founding, Sutherland had spent about a decade touring the state promoting mental health on behalf of a private foundation; during the 1950s and 1960s, he began "championing the role of private philanthropy in solving social problems" not only in Texas but across the Southwest region.[25] Sutherland took a broad view of philanthropy's role that reflected the expansive definition of mental health he and Ima Hogg had adopted for the Hogg Foundation. As Wayne Holtzman recalled, "It didn't matter whether you were a foundation that dealt with feeding elephants in the zoo or you were a foundation dealing with mental health or what. He wanted them all included."[26] The Conference of Southwest Foundations thus formed a "philanthropic community" that would further the trend of efficient, carefully targeted charity begun during the early twentieth century and would do so with the goal of supporting social needs and reforms in the Southwest region.

The individual who worked behind the scenes to transform Sutherland's vision for the Conference of Southwest Foundations into a reality for four decades was Maud Keeling, who had taken a position as Sutherland's assistant at the Hogg Foundation in 1945 as a twenty-one-year-old student of sociology and psychology at the University of Texas. Although she missed the first conference due to international travel, Keeling provided all the administrative, clerical, and research support for the conference out of the Hogg Foundation offices at the University of Texas. Even when her husband, a university professor, took a position in another state, Keeling continued to manage the conference's activities remotely. Her energetic networking

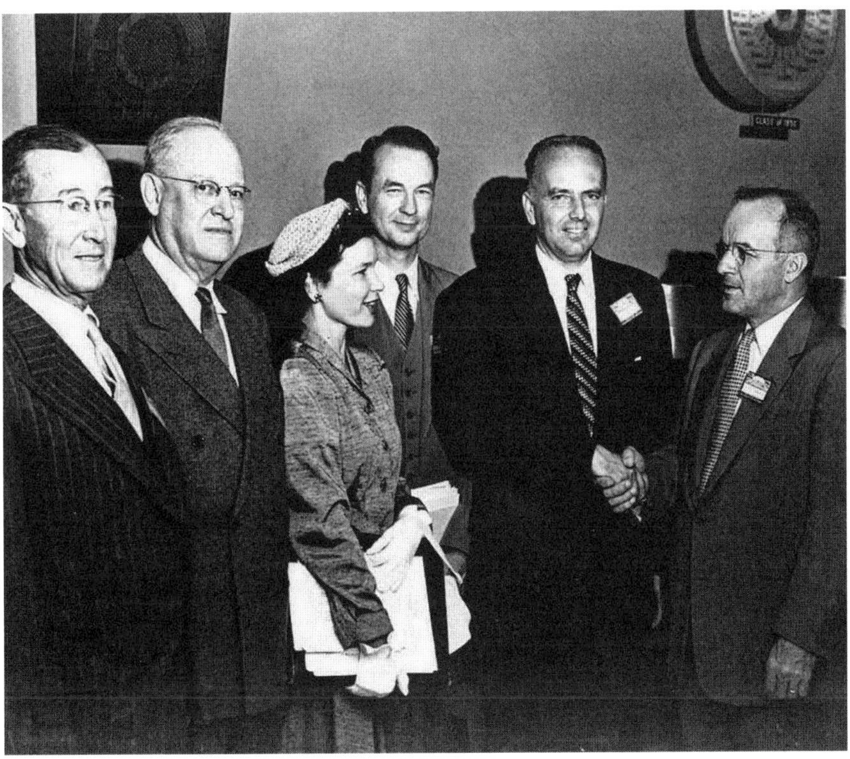

4.3. Maud Keeling (center, left) with Robert L. Sutherland, c. 1950. Courtesy of Philanthropy Southwest.

and management of the conference under such circumstances reflected her dedication to the conference's mission as well as her personal ties to Robert and Barbara Sutherland. As her successor and current executive director Lucille DiDomenico recalled, "The Conference files were in the trunk of her car. Wherever she moved, the Conference moved."[27] When her husband was killed in a boating accident several years later, Keeling returned to Texas to take a half-time position at the Driscoll Foundation in Corpus Christi, which then became the home office for the conference. Keeling's association with the conference spanned forty-six annual sessions, exceeding Sutherland's own career and lasting until 1996.[28]

Maud Keeling was one of several women who played prominent roles in the development of philanthropy and mental health during this period in Texas history—at a time when women rarely held such leadership positions. For women such as Ima Hogg, Mary Butt, and Margaret Scarborough, the emergence of organized philanthropy provided, in DiDomenico's words, "a leadership opportunity for women of wealth that many of the women took advantage of, because they would not have had the same opportunities to wield a similar kind of power in another walk of life."[29] At the Hogg Foundation, as noted in chapters 2 and 3, director Sutherland surrounded himself with female professionals led by Bert Kruger Smith and Bernice Milburn Moore. Although Smith and Moore were each married to a university professor and had taken positions at the Foundation as quasi-spousal hires that complied with the state's nepotism laws, each took on prominent roles delivering public lectures, consulting in communities, publishing research, and collaborating with the Conference of Southwest Foundations. DiDomenico speculated that Sutherland was personally comfortable working around female colleagues and that women were "moved by the cause of the foundation" to a greater extent than men during the middle decades of the twentieth century.[30] The Foundation even advocated for greater professional roles for women at times, such as in a 1963 pamphlet titled "Women View Their Working World," which was based on interviews with one hundred professional women. The author, psychology professor Ira Iscoe, concluded that it was "high time that the intellectual top level of American women put aside their guilt feelings and actually start to practice some of the independence of thought that their intense educational experience is supposed to provide. There is no telling how much frustration we actually bring about by imbuing a competent and potentially professional woman with the ideas of freedom and achievement and then bringing her face to face with social pressures which prevent her potential from coming to fruition."[31] Thus women from various backgrounds found avenues to leading roles through both the Hogg Foundation and the Conference of Southwest Foundations, and those organizations at times explicitly addressed issues of gender equality to the wider public. In many ways, however, Keeling exemplified some of the problems women still faced amid progress in the professions. According to both the leading history of the conference and current executive director DiDomenico, she was at times paid a clerical salary for a director's position and other times worked as essentially an unpaid volunteer.[32]

Nowhere was Keeling's importance to the conference more evident than in the organization's response to a growing backlash against philanthropic foundations during the 1950s and 1960s.[33] During the Cold War, anticommunist activists began to question the allegedly "subversive" role of private foundations whose activities were not subject to public scrutiny. Other critics contended that tax-exempt foundations were directing funds toward profit-generating and political ends, in violation of federal regulations. In 1962 these suspicions culminated with a Congressional investigation led by Representative Wright Patman of Texarkana, who chaired the House Small Business Committee. Decrying foundations as secretive "accumulators of massive wealth and power," Patman's committee uncovered some abuses and called for the removal of tax-exempt status and greater public oversight.[34] Foundation representatives countered that their contributions far outweighed the problems cited by Patman, a view echoed in a prominent news series in the *Fort Worth Star-Telegram* that was later reprinted as a mass-mailing pamphlet by the Conference of Southwest Foundations.[35] Nevertheless, the Treasury Department issued a report calling for more stringent regulations, and the Internal Revenue Service began conducting audits of several private foundations—particularly those that had not released annual reports or other forms of public disclosure. In 1967 the Conference of Southwest Foundations released a report, conducted by Keeling, of how regional foundations had responded to the criticism as well as to the increase in federal grants supporting some of the same types of issues that previously had been supported chiefly by private philanthropies. The report was supported by the Hogg Foundation under its Philanthropy in the Southwest program and drew on thirty interviews Keeling had conducted with foundation heads. She found that foundations had become more circumspect about supporting certain activities, such as college scholarships, that duplicated federal financial aid and had grown wary of publicizing their work.[36] However, this state of affairs proved temporary and did not halt the nearly 300 percent growth in foundation assets in the Southwest during the postwar era. Even the passage of the federal Tax Reform Act of 1969, which imposed restrictions on the financial and political activities of foundations and required them to pay an annual excise tax on investment income, did not dampen the continued growth of private philanthropy in the region.[37] As the leadership of the older family foundations began to pass to newer generations, and new startup foundations joined the conference, most members adhered to

Robert Sutherland's advice about how best to combat public concerns: use funds "for their intended purposes" and focus on "non-political, scientific, and humanitarian objectives."[38] Indeed, the conference embodied on a larger scale not only these values but also the Foundation's more pragmatic strategy of parlaying relatively small resources into significant social impact.

Thanks to its successful development of the conference, the Hogg Foundation was invited to assist with the inauguration of similar area foundation conferences in California, Michigan, and the Deep South.[39] In 1962, amid this developmental phase for the conference, the Hogg Foundation was designated by the Carnegie Foundation Library Center as one of seven Regional Foundation Libraries. Thus the Foundation's offices at the University of Texas became the repository for all records and information about philanthropy in the Southwest region.[40] The development of the Conference of Southwest Foundations provided the Hogg Foundation with a regional network of potential funding partners for mental health activities. Increasingly during this period, the Foundation began to turn its attention away from public education and toward applied research in mental health.

"We Know More Than We Put Into Practice": Mental Health Research

The emergence of the Conference of Southwest Foundations coincided with the development of the first significant research program at the Hogg Foundation. Between 1955 and 1976, the Foundation published a dozen research monographs on mental health and inaugurated the first mental health grants program that, by 1974, had evolved into an evaluation research grant program that would lay claim to being the first of its kind in Texas and the Southwest region.[41] The grants program provided seed money that enabled local and statewide mental health providers to compete for an expanding pool of federal grants. In 1951, the year before the program's launch, the National Institutes for Health awarded three hundred research grants for mental health, none of which went to Texas applicants; in 1958, the first year the Foundation tabulated such data, Texas had received seventeen research grant awards in mental health from the National Institutes of Health. Similarly, between 1955 and 1958, the Foundation awarded $80,000 in seed grants that resulted in over $1 million in federal grant awards in mental health from the National Institute for Mental Health, the National Science Foundation, and the federal Office of Education. The grantees were most often "intensive demonstration projects" led by faculty at the University of Texas collaborating with "other universities, clinics, mental hospitals, and state and community agencies."[42] In 1958 the Foundation declared that its "dual goals" were "to increase scientific knowledge and to see mental health principles at work in the schools, in community agencies, and in industry."[43]

The research program represented a departure from the Foundation's previous activities but one that its leadership embraced as an expansion of its historic mission to improve mental health for all Texans. In their frequent correspondence, Foundation director Sutherland and benefactor Ima Hogg discussed how the Foundation might expand its activities beyond public education and consulting. This conversation included topics such as how the Foundation could assist the University of Texas in launching its new School of Social Work; provide scholarships to students of psychology, psychiatry, and social work at several Texas colleges and universities; expand the Foundation's office space on the campus; and support various types of research in mental health.[44] The relationship between the pair had grown close by this time, which enabled Ima to persuade Sutherland to remain in the directorship despite offers from other universities. "The Foundation has begun to mean 'Robert Sutherland,'" she wrote in 1950, "and I'm happy you are staying with it despite such flattering offers!"[45] In 1952 Ima decided to sell the remainder of her ownership in the Varner Company—which managed the family's oil-rich property holdings in East Texas—to the University of Texas, with a directive that the proceeds be added to the Hogg Foundation's endowment. On June 30, 1952, the Hogg family and its attorneys met in Houston with Dudley K. Woodward, the chairman of the Board of Regents. At the meeting, Ima expressed her intent that "the real estate purchased for the Hogg Foundation will accrue richly to the benefit of the Foundation."[46] The transaction was officially recorded at the July 1952 meeting of the Board of Regents, at a price of $6.5 million, which more than tripled the Hogg Foundation's existing endowment of about $3 million.[47] However, the Foundation saw no immediate increase in its operating budget. In her letter to Chairman Woodward acknowledging the transaction, Ima had expressed concern that many of the newer regents and university officials did not understand "the objectives and activities" of the Foundation. "The members of our family have taken, and shall continue to take, a deep interest in the success of this work for mental health in Texas," she warned.[48] When the university failed to increase the Foundation's budget in 1953–54, Ima responded by summoning the Board of Regents to her home in Houston for a special meeting in October 1953. Joining the gathering were University of Texas administrators, Hogg family members, and Texas business heads (several of whom were leading figures at the Texas Conference of Foundations and Trusts Funds). At this meeting, Ima and Sutherland presented the Foundation's achievements and its future plans, noting the Foundation's unique status as a private endowment managed by a public university board and moreover the single largest endowment managed by the university—a not-too-subtle suggestion that the family might rescind the award should the university fail to follow its wishes in supporting the Foundation. Other prominent speakers reinforced this message by touting the Foundation's good works.[49]

One possible reason for the slow application of new funds to the Foundation's budget was that the University of Texas was in the midst of a leadership transition. In 1953 the new president, Logan Wilson, took office with a mandate to expand dramatically the research profile of the university. As Sutherland would later recount, Wilson and the board put "considerable pressure" on the Foundation to devote significant resources to support faculty research and the expansion of clinical research facilities at the university.[50] In meetings with the Foundation staff, Wilson "indicated . . . that he was particularly interested in the work of the Hogg Foundation tying in closely with the main branch of the University in its research and teaching programs, as well as the work which it has been doing throughout the state on a broader base. Dr. Wilson had expressed great interest in emphasis upon research in the field of human relations and human behavior."[51]

Wilson's interests dovetailed in some ways with those of the Foundation itself, although there were some key differences. With Ima's backing, director Sutherland had established several external advisory boards that began meeting in 1950 to help the Foundation map out a new direction in anticipation of increased budget resources. Sutherland met with advisory groups from the Texas Neuropsychiatric Association, the Texas Psychological Association, and the Texas Social Welfare Association during the early 1950s. Even before the arrival of President Wilson, the deliberations of these panels focused almost exclusively on research, and particularly on the types of research that were most appropriate for the Foundation's mission and resources. Suggestions included more surveys of the needs in various communities and evaluative research on community and industrial mental health programs.[52] However, the focus on research heightened for these panels after the increase in the Hogg Foundation endowment and the arrival of President Wilson. In January 1954, Sutherland summarized the feedback provided by the advisory boards. The consensus was that the Foundation should engage largely in "evaluative" and "action" research; essentially the panels advised a focus on applied rather than basic research. This emphasis squared with the Foundation's mission as well as Ima Hogg's often-stated viewpoint that "we already know so much more than we put into practice" regarding mental health. Indeed, upon reviewing Sutherland's initial research program policy, which focused on applied research, Ima declared that she was "glad research is part of the program."[53] Sutherland, however, worried that it was at odds with President Wilson's "philosophy that ideas should be propagated at the University of Texas and disseminated out from there, rather than the gathering of ideas from communities and bringing them together at the University for the use of others."[54] This tension between basic and applied research would continue through the early years of the Foundation's research program.

Finally, in July 1953, separate conferences between the Foundation, its various advisory boards, and President Wilson produced an agreed-upon outline of the scope, character, and structure of the new research program. The outcome was a statement of "principles as a partial indication of present trends in the Foundation program." The Foundation was to embark upon the following plans: secure "additional professional staff so as to give closer supervision to projects financed or co-financed by the Foundation," "aid in the establishment of a social science research institute" that could help with "screening and supervising certain projects," and "maintain at least a loose control over the projects" instead of "making blanket grants to other organizations." While the proposed research institute never came into being, the Foundation did begin awarding small research grants at the University of Texas in 1954–55.[55] During that time, the Foundation's annual operating budget more than doubled from $130,000 to $345,000.[56]

The new research program was placed in the hands of Wayne Holtzman, who became Associate Director for Research in 1954. A native of Chicago, Holtzman had earned an undergraduate degree in chemistry at Northwestern University prior to joining the Navy in 1944. While serving as an anti-aircraft gunnery officer on the *U.S.S. Iowa*, and later as a communications aide for the Third and Fifth Fleet, Holtzman "became interested in why some of the men in the Navy were breaking down under stress, whereas others weren't."[57] Holtzman returned to Chicago with an interest in psychology and psychiatry; he earned a master's degree at Northwestern and later completed a doctoral degree in psychology at Stanford University in 1949. That same year, he accepted a faculty position in the psychology department at the University of Texas, which at the time was a small but growing program. One of "the first people" he met was Robert Sutherland, who enlisted Holtzman as one of the Hogg Foundation's circuit riders speaking to groups around the state about mental hygiene. By 1954 the relationship between Holtzman and Sutherland had grown close enough that Holtzman was entrusted to serve as acting director while Sutherland traveled overseas; in Holtzman's recounting, Sutherland was his "mentor in many ways."[58] Although they arrived at the Foundation with formal training in the distinct disciplines of sociology and psychology, Sutherland and Holtzman appear to have agreed generally about approaching mental health from multidisciplinary and interdisciplinary perspectives. In this respect, they reflected the prevalent currents in many of the social and behavioral sciences at that time, when "culture and personality" researchers such as Harry Stack Sullivan, Karen Horney, and Adolph Meyer (who had served on the Foundation's initial advisory board in 1940–41) combined the insights of psychiatry, psychology, sociology, and anthropology in exploring elements of human personality.[59] The pair collaborated well, and thus Holtzman became the obvious choice to lead the research program that Logan Wilson envisioned for the Foundation.

The full scope and direction of the research program was agreed upon at an advisory conference that took place in Dallas in April 1955. Participants included Ima Hogg, Robert Sutherland, Wayne Holtzman, Logan Wilson, and members of the Foundation's Citizen Advisory Board led by psychiatrist William Menninger. Wilson articulated his vision that a regional university such as the University of Texas could grow into a major research institution only by nurturing "peaks of excellence" into programs of national and international renown.[60] In his view, the Foundation could best serve that role by "develop[ing] a program of research and publication which will have national significance."[61]

> Dr. Wilson further stressed the significance of the Foundation's relationship to the University. Obviously, the Foundation's program will enrich the teaching and research activities of the various departments and branches . . . related to the field of mental health, but also in carrying out its obligation of service to the communities of the state [it] . . . can involve University staff members and students in the planning and execution of the projects.
>
> Dr. Wilson recommended that the Foundation concentrate its work in a limited number of fields in order to make a substantial contribution. He said that the program did not need to be conceived as "ivory tower." In fact, even the research can include field studies whose findings will be of value to other phases of the program.[62]

Advisory committee member Loyd Rowland, architect of the Pierre the Pelican campaign, suggested that the Foundation should "finance pilot projects" in mental health because the needs surrounding mental health and mental illness were "too gigantic for the Foundation to approach directly." Menninger concurred, urging that the Foundation sponsor demonstration projects to "awaken the public" to the needs of people with mental illness.[63] Shortly after that meeting, Sutherland informed the members of the various advisory committees that those bodies were being dissolved. He also announced the inauguration of the research program, headed by Holtzman, with a staff that included Bernice Milburn Moore, Bert Kruger Smith, and others, who would consult individually with now-former advisory committee members.[64] That summer, Sutherland convened a staff meeting at the Foundation offices to lay final plans for the research program, which he described as a "considerable change in policy, program, and procedures." The plan for the upcoming

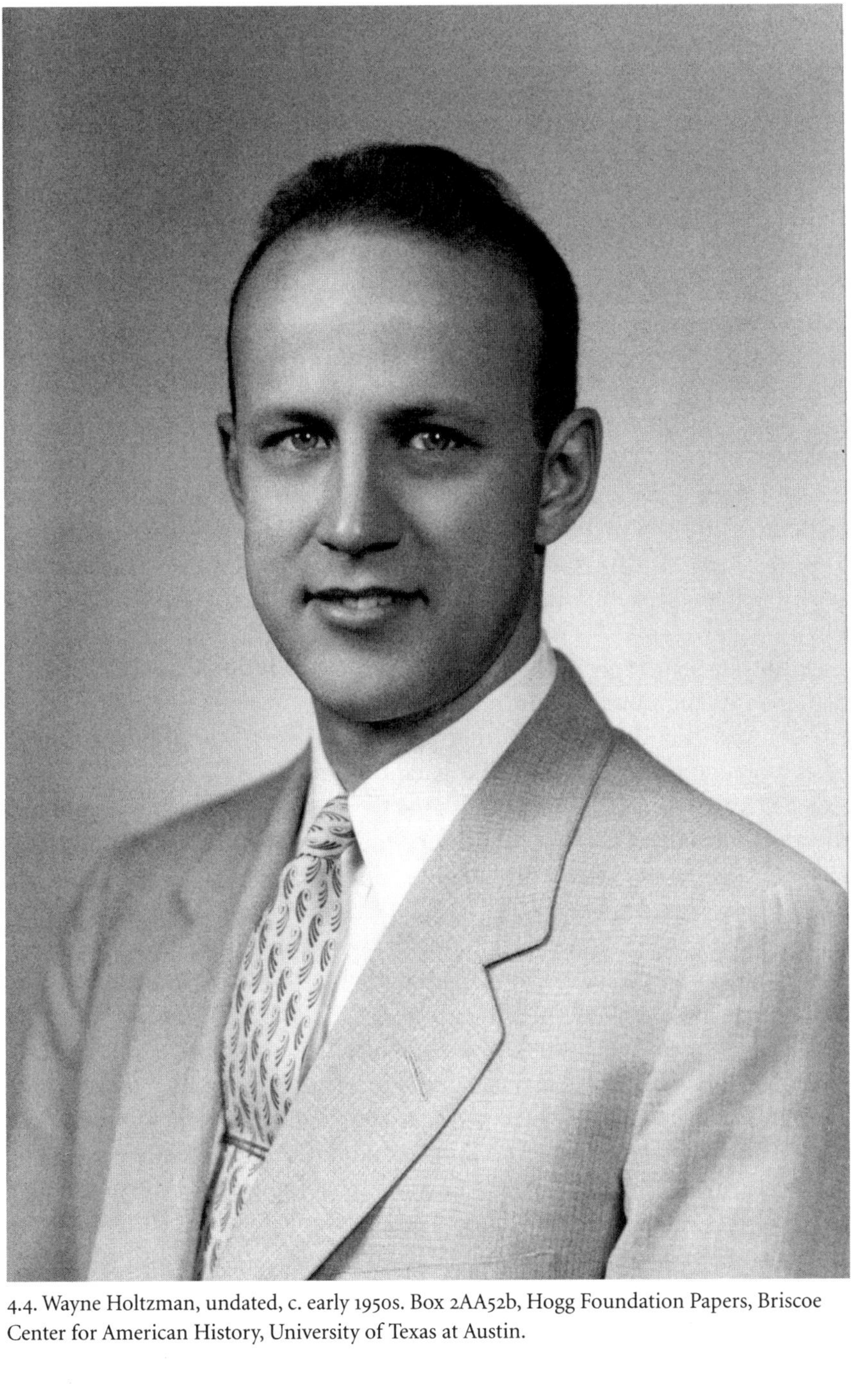

4.4. Wayne Holtzman, undated, c. early 1950s. Box 2AA52b, Hogg Foundation Papers, Briscoe Center for American History, University of Texas at Austin.

year was "based upon a budget of $300,000 a year, one-half of which will be ear-marked for research and research publications."[65] The allotment of half the budget for research became established practice for the next several years.[66] In place of visiting lectures at an "elementary instructional level," the Foundation provided expert consultation for pilot programs in mental health that could offer professional development opportunities for junior faculty or graduate students and that could provide opportunities for evaluative research.[67] In addition, as Holtzman recounted, "the idea was to . . . have starter grants to places where there was a promising young investigator who needed a little bit of something to get him up and going so he could get a larger grant from the National Institute of Mental Health or the National Science Foundation." The vast majority of these grants were awarded to faculty at the University of Texas. In 1958 the Foundation reported that it was supporting "sixteen major areas of graduate research activity" ranging from "biochemistry and neurophysiology to sociology and education, from laboratory studies to field research involving entire communities. In some of these sixteen areas, the Foundation has played a supportive role by facilitating the well-developed plans of one or more individuals. In most, however, the Foundation and its consultants have taken an active leadership role in bringing together the interests and skills of men from different University departments."[68] The Foundation also was providing support to the state hospitals and special schools in "planning small projects which would demonstrate the value of more adequate support" from the state. The report concluded by boldly predicting that the Foundation's "stimulus to graduate education and basic research will constantly increase."[69]

The Foundation collaborated with the University of Texas Press to publish the more substantial projects funded under the research grants program. This Hogg Foundation Research Monograph Series produced a dozen books over a nearly two-decade period (1958–76). Edited by Holtzman, the series began with *Tornadoes Over Texas* (1958), a study by sociologist Harry Estill Moore of the community response to tornadoes that struck Waco and San Angelo, in the "tornado alley" region of north central Texas, on the same day in May 1953.[70] The first tornado struck in a residential area of San Angelo in the early afternoon, killing 11 and injuring 159 persons; later that evening, another tornado touched down in downtown Waco, demolishing or structurally damaging 572 buildings, killing 114, and injuring 1,097. Combined damages fell just short of $60 million.[71] "Among the first and most important contributions to the modern study of disaster," Moore's study, conducted during the two years immediately following these disasters, is today considered a classic sociological study of natural disasters.[72] "[E]ach of its 14 empirical chapters," asserts one recent assessment, "either spawned a new line of inquiry or established a precedent for what to examine in a field study of disaster."[73] *Tornadoes Over*

Texas relied on organizational records, newspaper accounts, household surveys, and in-depth interviews with disaster victims. It explored the damage and recovery from material and mental health perspectives, focusing especially on the plight of the elderly and on racial differences in the experience of disaster and relief efforts. Noting that the black and white populations of Waco lived "on opposite sides of a cultural fault line," Moore demonstrated disparities in impact and relief support between black and white families.[74] Finally, Moore described the emotional responses of disaster victims and noted ways in which local and federal officials could address their psychological as well as material needs. The study continues to be cited as a foundational text in the study of disasters and disaster relief.[75]

In the wake of *Tornadoes Over Texas*, the Foundation decided to seek more external guidance in its approach to research, as well as other important areas such as public policy, grant-making, and professional development. At two key junctures in its history, the Foundation convened ad hoc advisory boards: during the Foundation's formation in 1940–41 and during the development of its research program in 1949–54. Now, the Foundation opted to form a permanent National Advisory Council (NAC) comprised of prominent mental health experts with reputations at the state and national levels. The first NAC met in May 1959 and included Joseph Bobbitt, assistant director of the National Institute of Mental Health; prominent child psychologist William Adamson; and Ralph Tyler, director of the Center for Advanced Study in the Behavioral Sciences. These annual meetings, which continue to this day, have provided the Foundation with valuable input and, as we shall see, at times pushed the Foundation to keep pace with national trends in mental health. At the initial NAC gathering, the discussion focused entirely on the scope and focus of the Foundation's still-new research program, with a particular discussion of how best to balance "competing mandates for scholarly attainment on the one hand and for community service on the other."[76]

These "competing mandates" would be reflected in subsequent publications, which ranged across various topics and disciplines, even as they made significant contributions to their respective fields. In 1961 associate director Holtzman published an inkblot perception and personality test that addressed some shortcomings in the Rorschach inkblot test. The Holtzman Inkblot Technique would go on to be widely used by psychologists and psychiatrists in a variety of settings, in both the United States and Mexico.[77] The third book in the series was an anthology of research papers given at a symposium held at the Texas Medical Center in Houston. Titled *Electrical Stimulation of the Brain: An Interdisciplinary Survey of Neurobehavioral Integrative Systems*, the volume's contributors addressed "the problem of 'higher order' behaviors usually subsumed under such psychological rubrics as perception, learning, emotion, and motivation."[78] However, such highly specialized volumes proved to be the exception rather than the rule for the research series. Far more typical was the project that arose from a community mental health demonstration project—in other words, more "applied" than "basic" mental health research. Subsequent book-length studies in the 1960s focused on a parent education program in Austin, mental health services provided at an old-age residential housing project in San Antonio, and a mental health program developed for Anglo and Mexican populations in Hidalgo County in south Texas.[79]

The research program elicited some controversy, both internally and externally. Within the Foundation, it appears that the main benefactor, Ima Hogg, became concerned about what she perceived as a divergence from the statewide, public mission to "improve mental health for the people of Texas." More prominent, however, was the emergence of a small but vocal "anti-mental health" movement from the political right, which characterized the Foundation's research efforts as tied to Communist subversion.

"An Evil and Subversive Thing": The Anti-Mental Health Movement

In its first two decades, the Hogg Foundation not only became closely identified with mental health in the broadest sense but also associated itself with specific programs such as community-based mental health services, guidance counseling programs in public schools, parenting advice informed by mental health principles, and encouragement of more humane treatment of people with mental illness in institutional settings. The Foundation also developed collaborations with business leaders to introduce mental health reforms into the workplace. Even while participating in public policy debates, however, the Foundation avoided being drawn into partisan political activity. Nevertheless, as we have seen, at times political appointees such as University of Texas regents, or elected officials, voiced criticisms of mental health generally, and its associated academic disciplines specifically. These suspicions spiked in an "anti-mental health" movement that coalesced on the radical right during the late 1950s and early 1960s. This movement drew its inspiration from the Second Red Scare, a short but intense period of panic about Communists and "fellow travelers" that supposedly had infiltrated public and private organizations in American society. Powerful national officials such as Richard Nixon and Joseph McCarthy mounted well-publicized investigations of federal agencies, while the House Un-American Activities Committee held high-profile hearings investigating Communist subversion in the motion-picture industry. Meanwhile, at the state and local levels, investigations targeted public schools, colleges and universities, and even public libraries for "reducator" teachers or materials that could be deemed critical of American politics and society.[80] By the late 1950s, the Red Scare had begun to subside in intensity, but in its wake, organizations sprang up on the political fringes that continued and expanded on its activities. Some of these organizations were national in scope, such as the John Birch Society, while others were regional or even statewide or local in focus. National circulation magazines such as the *National Review* and regionally distributed talk-radio programs served as venues for this conservative political movement. In his famous 1964 essay "The Paranoid Style in American Politics," historian Richard Hofstadter identified this movement's chief enemies: shadowy, vaguely defined conspiracies of perceived elites, associated with established cultural, social, or political institutions.[81] Led by academic experts, large universities, private philanthropies, and government agencies, mental health would prove to be an ideal target for this movement.

Mental health indeed found itself in the radical right's cross-hairs by the late 1950s. In the forefront was Matt Cvetic, a former agent at the Federal Bureau of Investigation who had spent nine years in the 1940s working undercover in the American Communist Party. His experiences became the subject of a series of articles in the *Saturday Evening Post* and in the 1951 motion picture *I Was a Communist for the FBI*. In a 1959 article published in *American Mercury* magazine, Cvetic recounted that during his undercover work he had learned of the existence of a "professional unit" in the Communist Party, comprised of "psychiatrists, psychologists, medical doctors and social, health and welfare workers." Members of this unit, he warned, were working as "thought control agents . . . within the mental health and welfare programs of our nation."[82] Cvetic's warnings were circulated in Texas by a loose-knit group of conservative activists, led by Dan Smoot, another former FBI agent based in Dallas, who left the agency in 1951 to become a political activist. Starting in the mid-1950s, Smoot began publishing a weekly newsletter titled *The Dan Smoot Report* and hosting a weekly talk-radio program. At its peak circulation, Smoot's newsletter had more than 30,000 subscribers.[83] One of Smoot's first major campaigns concerned a federal bill, the Alaska Mental Health Act of 1956, which attempted to put aside 1 million acres of federal land and provide funds for the establishment of mental health clinics and hospitals in the then-territory of Alaska. Smoot and other conservative activists labeled this law the "Siberia Bill" and alleged that it was a conspiracy to establish prison camps where psychiatrists would engage in "brainwashing" American citizens.[84] They also denounced philanthropic foundations that supported such activities, such as the Ford Foundation, as having been infiltrated with subversives. In Texas, conservative activists attempted—and nearly succeeded—in getting a bill passed by the legislature that would have removed the state requirement that all public schools maintain guidance counseling programs, which they viewed as a "guise for mental health programs" and "the strangle-hold of progressive educationalists in the state of Texas."[85]

The project that attracted attention to the Hogg Foundation was the research eventually published in 1965 as *Tomorrow's Parents: A Study of Youth and Their Families* as part of the Foundation's research monograph series. The data for this book was gathered during the Texas Cooperative Youth Study, a survey of nearly 13,000 high school students in Texas, conducted by a team of about thirty researchers. The survey protocol was developed by Wayne Holtzman and Bernice Milburn Moore, both Hogg Foundation researchers, and Carson McGuire, a University of Texas professor of human relations. McGuire's area of expertise was adolescent development; in 1950 he had joined Erik Erikson on a panel titled "Crucial Conflicts in Personality Development in Youth and Young Adulthood" at the Midcentury White House Conference on Children and Youth.[86] Erikson's influential concepts of adolescent "identity crisis" and identity formation helped shape the survey questions of the Texas Cooperative Youth Study. Based on a psychological attitude scales model, the survey's questions were broken into fourteen categories measuring young people's feelings about American society, schoolteachers, parents, and peers. Additionally, the scales attempted to tease out personal characteristics such as authoritarianism, conformity, level of self-esteem, and resentment of "dependency" upon adults. Holtzman and Moore then correlated the results with social survey data on the family and household, a method common in postwar social scientific research that sought to explain how different individuals and groups were adjusting to their particular social structure. Results that showed a significant disparity between attitudes and circumstances led many researchers in this period to draw conclusions about emotional "maladjustment."

The main thesis of *Tomorrow's Parents* was that families "remain the major agents in the socialization of the young and . . . the paramount institution in society for the transmission of culture."[87] While this statement seemed hardly controversial, it was accompanied by data tables that suggested children with two working parents suffered no more than those headed by a male breadwinner. Moreover, the study concluded that the most "healthy" teenagers came from families in which both parents had achieved high levels of education and occupational status. Supporters of a "traditional" family structure with a male breadwinner and a female homemaker might find little support in such a conclusion. The study also included surveys of African American and Mexican American teenagers, who generally expressed pessimistic expectations for adulthood, negative views of society, and suspicions of adult authority. According to the study, these teenagers were more likely to come from single-parent households with adults who had lower educational attainment. The study concluded that the attitudes reflected some "maladjustment" to societal norms but also resulted from racial discrimination, particularly school segregation, whose eradication the study characterized as "well under way."[88]

These relatively tame statements about racial minorities and family norms emerged from survey questionnaires that had struck a nerve with anti-mental health activists around the state. Perhaps the fiercest controversy erupted in Houston, where a version of the Texas Cooperative Youth Study was conducted during the spring of 1959 with the approval of the Houston Independent School District. The Houston Youth Study, as the survey was billed, did not enjoy unanimous support. The Houston school board was divided over the study, with one faction of so-called Minute Women bitterly opposing the study. As chronicled by historian Don Carleton, the Minute Women represented an ultra-conservative, anticommunist group that had controlled the board for much of the 1950s, mounting purges of "subversive" teachers and textbooks. By the time of the Houston Youth Study, however, the board was joined by its first African American member, Hattie Mae White, and was grappling with school desegregation along with other hot-button issues. The backdrop thus was one of political division, with one side closely attuned to anything that smacked of "radical" or "subversive" activity: for example, a survey questionnaire circulated among high school students that included questions about sex, race relations, social class, adult authority, and patriotism.[89] In addition, the survey's authorship evoked several conservative bogeymen: the outside agitator, the academic expert, and the philanthropic foundation. The official sponsors of the Houston Youth Study were the American Institute of Research housed at the University of Pittsburgh, the Hogg Foundation for Mental Health, and the Child Welfare Section of the Houston Community Council.[90]

Perhaps recognizing these potential land mines, the cover page of the study began with a statement of purpose that cited "the great loss to society of the countless thousands of youth who fail . . . to realize their full capacities for learning and achievement." The study promised to assist local authorities in "combat[ing] juvenile delinquency on a community-wide level" while also addressing questions to both "gifted youth" and "delinquents." Furthermore, the study's questions were developed for youth irrespective of "national or regional borders" and were not intended to target purely local or regional mores. Last, student test-takers found in their booklets repeated assurances of anonymity.[91] The survey included only one section testing scholarly aptitude: a vocabulary quiz. The American Institute of Research contributed two sections, one in which students listed their preferred occupations and leisure activities and another that measured personality scales for desirable traits such as assertiveness, sociability, and self-reliance. None of this material drew public criticism. The Youth Attitude Scales section, contributed by the Hogg Foundation, drew the lion's share of attention. Researchers had viewed this section as potentially shedding unique light on student struggles to make good grades, while opponents singled out the intrusiveness of the questions. Defenders of the study explained the ten attitude scales based on student responses to "personal" statements as responding to "the urgent need for more scientifically sound information dealing with how youth feel about themselves, their families, schools, and associates."[92]

Some objections to the survey were expressed in common-sense language. For example, the booklet required significant school time to complete; indeed, the vocabulary section alone included more than three hundred multiple-choice questions. The student information section asked for schedule data on family income, school attendance, religion, housing, gender, age, household size, race and ethnicity, health, and future plans for education. The Youth Attitude Scales section asked students to agree or disagree with a series of statements, a sampling of which includes

> Most teachers are too rigid and narrow-minded.
>
> A person should insist on his rights no matter what.
>
> In spite of what some people say, life for the average person is getting worse, not better.
>
> We ought to worry about our own country and let the rest of the world take care of itself.
>
> Housekeeping in our house is disorderly.
>
> My parents rarely go to church.
>
> I am never able to discuss problems confidentially with either of my parents.[93]

The possible implications of such questions aroused angry objections, particularly to a perceived invasion of privacy. "It seems that no family skeleton is safe from the sociologists anymore," sighed an editorial in the *Houston Chronicle*.[94] Even more explosive were the questions about racial and ethnic prejudice included in the Youth Attitude Scales section. These entries asked students to describe their feelings toward "Anglos and Latins," "Negroes," the elderly, and people with mental illness or with disabilities.[95] Such questions recalled another association that surely played into the minds of school board members—that of mental health with racial integration. Testimony from psychologists, led by Kenneth Clark, had demonstrated the emotional damage caused by segregated schooling and played a critical role in the landmark Supreme Court ruling in *Brown v. Board of Education* (1954). For many Southern whites who defended the Jim Crow system of racial segregation and discrimination, the professions most closely associated with mental health had deemed their way of life to be a form of mental illness. Indeed, the lone board member to cast a vote in support of the study was its only African American member, Hattie Mae White, who frequently found herself in the minority until the board's composition began to change in the mid-1960s.[96]

Opposition to the Houston Youth Study reached a boiling point in June 1959, when some parents organized against the release of the test data. They appeared at a televised session of the school board, where they joined conservative members in denouncing the survey and demanding the destruction of its results.[97] Finally, the Houston Youth Study's local chairperson bowed to pressure by burning the test data in front of reporters, an act that was later likened to a "book-burning" by one child welfare expert.[98] Conservatives, for their part, decried the survey as "an evil and subversive thing," with one newsletter dubbing the Hogg Foundation "an institution noted for its assistance to left-wing movements."[99] The Houston Community Council, meanwhile, was torn with factional struggle after the controversy broke out. Its wealthy benefactors and their wives (some of whom sat on the school board) opposed the release of the test data, which had been collected by the social workers, academics, and clinicians who served on the Council's Child Welfare section. A distraught Ima Hogg wrote from Houston that she was "awfully sorry that things have not gone the way they should." She reminded director Sutherland that she had "thought Houston was not the right place" for such a study: "There are certain peculiar conditions here so that almost any worthy effort is stymied before it starts!"[100]

The Houston Youth Study affair shined a spotlight on the Hogg Foundation for anti-mental health activists. In February 1960, director Sutherland and associate director Holtzman examined the allegation that the Ford Foundation's 1959 annual report showed Communist influence when compared with its 1950 report. Characterizing the suggestion as "crackpot," Holtzman found "very little" substance to the charges. "I don't think there's anything on God's green Earth that [the Ford Foundation] could do to eliminate such hostility from . . . misguided outgroups like this one," he lamented, warning that "nevertheless we ought to keep such quasi-paranoid attacks in mind as we go about our own business."[101] In March 1961, amid a push to legislate against guidance counseling programs, state Senator Dorsey B. Hardeman of San Angelo, who had been critical of mental health activity previously (see chapter 3), complained about questionnaires sent home with students "at the behest of tax-exempt foundations, organizations and self-styled researchers" that sought "information about delicate and highly personal private family matters."[102] One newsletter listed the supporters of guidance counseling in language that evoked not only far-right opposition to mental health but also criticisms of private foundations:

> [T]he foggy advocates of federal control, the socialists, the do-gooders, and especially the Hogg Foundation for Mental Health—that perversion of a great Texas family tradition through the ill-advised, tax-exempt use of its own fortune. This meddlesome, misguided outfit, long aggressive in sinister mental health intrusions into private affairs, is pushing seminars at chosen colleges throughout the state . . . with six-week courses for pseudo-psychiatrists, hand-picked in accord with U.S. Office of Education "criteria," and financed individually by federal grants.[103]

Soon after, in April 1961, conservative commentator Dan Smoot launched an attack on the Hogg Foundation by name, blaming it for the "psychoanalysis of children and guidance of their future careers."[104] He also "singled out for intensive treatment" the Foundation's role in the Houston Youth Study. In the Houston area, Smoot's audience included Ima Hogg, members of the Board of Regents, and members of the Mental Health Association of Houston, several of whom contacted director Sutherland to express alarm. Of the Houston Youth Study, Ima Hogg recounted that she "did not like many of the questions on the instrument, thought that it should not have been given to the children, and was glad that the results were burned."[105] This episode would cause Ima to rethink the research program to some extent. In November 1961, she participated in a recorded interview with director Sutherland in which she spelled out her concerns, repeating her oft-stated injunction that "we know more than we put into practice."[106] While Ima continued to defer to the Foundation staff, she reiterated her view that its support for research should be guided by its results for the state and the public. Of what might be called "basic" research, she felt that "a great deal of research can be done in the medical schools because they are there together and are prepared."[107] The episode led to a meeting the following spring with the Board of Regents at Ima's home in Houston, where Sutherland reassured members about the Foundation's activities. The meeting was a positive one, during which Ima urged the Foundation to award "more fellowships" because "we need more people who are trained to carry on this program."[108] In a subsequent letter to University of Texas President Harry Ransom, Ima wrote that she had "been gratified by the manner in which my brother's bequest has been handled. I feel increasingly confident that the Mental Health program, such as we have outlined, would come as near as anything I can imagine being what my brother would endorse."[109]

The Foundation also sought guidance on the controversy from its National Advisory Council at its June 1961 meeting, which held an open-ended discussion about the political pitfalls confronting mental health research, particularly at universities.[110] Holtzman noted that some academics around the state had set up private research entities outside the university structure as a way to evade pressures from conservative political appointees and elected officials. He also observed that some campus administrators would oppose projects merely because the Foundation's name was attached to it—as a result of the negative publicity in conservative media. As an example, he pointed to a proposed attitude survey of students at Baylor University, a private Baptist institution, regarding religion and race relations; Holtzman feared that the Foundation would be held up as a "scapegoat" at the first sign of controversy. "The Houston Youth Study is a good case in point here," Holtzman stated, where "a small, militant, self-appointed minority decides that this is an evil that is being perpetuated as part of the grand conspiracy." The group concluded that the Foundation would need to exercise more caution in administering such surveys, because of "the line that Dan Smoot . . . and the John Birch Society and the Minute Women have taken, that any kind of social science study or activity, like counseling, psychiatry or research which has personal questions about your family life, is invading privacy, the next step is brain washing, and that's preparatory to implanting Communistic ideals." Even though, as Sutherland put it, this reaction was "almost accidental" in its "focus on mental health," the problem confronting the Foundation was that "in every Texas community and college now there are these people who would seize any statement, say from a questionnaire or from an interview procedure, take it back to their parents, who may be members of the John Birch Society." Bernice Moore worried that mental health proponents might "start to withdraw from the field of mental health and retreat literally into the generally safe area of mental illness."

As we shall see in the next chapter, no such retreat took place; in fact, the opposite occurred. The postwar era began with the Foundation sponsoring community mental health activities, such as the Pierre the Pelican parenting endeavor, on a relatively small scale due to limited resources. Such programs piloted new mental health services while also including elements of an evaluation research component. A confluence of events provided the Foundation with an opportunity to expand this program: expanded awareness of mental health around the state of Texas, the development of a coherent regional network of foundations, an infusion of new financial resources, and a push from the University of Texas to make research more of a priority. However, the new research program ran afoul of a political movement on the right that viewed social science and mental health with suspicion—particularly when it came from large, organized institutions. Indeed, one wonders how opponents of mental health would have reacted to the Pierre the Pelican campaign, which reached into one of the most private of activities—the parental care of infants and children. Although this movement's impact was somewhat disproportionate to its apparent size, it managed to produce a chilling effect on mental health research that would prove to be temporary. The social and political currents that nurtured the anti-mental health movement took a dramatic turn in the 1960s, as did the field of mental health itself, as we shall see in the next chapter.

5

"This Most Urgent of All Health Problems"

Community Mental Health in the 1960s

In February 1967, a letter arrived at the Hogg Foundation offices for Bert Kruger Smith, from "the mother of a 20 year old boy who has been mentally ill for over 5 years now." The writer of the letter was exasperated with her inability to locate assistance, having sent her son to "different hospitals, halfway-houses, etc., all private and out of state because of the poor facilities here." The expense of these measures had exhausted her financial resources, leaving the family with no other choice but "to bring him back to what Texas has to offer." The mother wrote to Smith seeking guidance while expressing her support for ongoing proposals to expand community-based mental health services: "Therefore I am keenly interested to do all I can to help push Mr. Connally's proposals. Can you help me and guide me as to what I can do as an individual?"[1] Coming two years after the passage of the landmark Texas Mental Health and Mental Retardation Act (H.B. 3, 1965), which created the Texas Department of Mental Health and Mental Retardation (TDMHMR), such a letter revealed the ongoing gap between promise and reality that often governed mental health reform. Throughout the postwar era, proponents of mental health reform in Texas advocated for the replacement of institutional facilities such as mental hospitals with community-based services. These new services were provided through new, smaller-scale facilities such as outpatient clinics, group homes, and halfway houses. In addition, reformers envisioned the expansion or introduction of mental health services within existing social institutions such as public schools, workplaces, and churches. As we have seen, Texas had taken halting steps toward realizing these reformist visions in the post–World War II era. The state legislature had created an agency devoted to improving its system of mental hospitals and special schools, expanded its resources devoted to supporting those institutions, and provided for an influx of psychiatric and psychological expertise to oversee improvements to mental health programming. In addition, the state Department of Health had established a Division of Mental Health to provide educational support to public schools and other organizations, albeit on a very limited basis. Although these steps were significant, they focused almost entirely on large institutions and had done little to address reformers' aspirations for community-based services. By the early 1960s, only a handful of mental health clinics operated in the state, and most of those were child guidance clinics that had opened before or immediately after World War II. Although it had voiced support for such clinics, the Board of Texas State Hospitals and Special Schools (BTSHSS) had managed to open only four of them during the 1950s, in San Antonio, Harlingen, Fort Worth, and Dallas.

The image of inertia on this front would prove to be deceptive. In addition to the changes underway in Texas, proponents of mental health were making major strides at the national level. Most significant was the passage of the Mental Health Study Act in 1955, which created the Joint Commission on Mental Illness and Health (JCMIH) as a nongovernmental body that was nevertheless endorsed by the federal government and received some federal funding. Led by members of the American Psychiatric Association and American Medical Association, the JCMIH emerged from planning sessions involving representatives of thirty-six national organizations. It was interdisciplinary in character, with physicians, psychiatrists, psychologists, sociologists, psychiatric social workers, nurses, as well as a public relations specialist. The director of the JCMIH was Jack Ewalt, formerly of the University of Texas Medical Branch in Galveston and at the time commissioner of mental health for the state of Massachusetts. The JCMIH was tasked with producing scholarly research that would define the prevalence of types of mental illness and making policy recommendations regarding the institutional and non-institutional services available for the prevention and treatment of mental illness. After producing ten individual studies, the JCMIH concluded its work in March 1961 with the publication of its final report, titled *Action for Mental Health.*[2]

The timing of the report's release coincided with the inauguration of John F. Kennedy, whose administration was expected to be more sympathetic than that of his predecessor to a proposal for sweeping change to the nation's social policies. *Action for Mental Health* summarized the "unmet needs" of people with mental illness and made four major recommendations: larger investments in basic research, an expansion of trained workers and services, education of the public about mental health and mental illness, and a massive increase in federal funding that would support a tripling of expenditures for mental health services over the subsequent ten years. Perhaps the most revolutionary element of the report was that it mapped out a national program with the community mental health clinic at its center. The JCMIH called for the establishment of one clinic for every 50,000 people while also recommending a halt to the construction of any state mental hospital with more than 1,000 beds and a reconversion of existing hospitals into centers strictly for individuals who truly required long-term care. Citing a time of "new hope," the report challenged legislators to "make history by adopting a new policy of action for mental health."[3]

Two years later, the federal government enacted the Community Mental Health Centers Act of 1963, which authorized $150 million in grants toward the construction of clinics between the years 1965 and 1967. Focused entirely on community clinics, the law went even further than had the JCMIH in emphasizing treatment in a community over a hospital setting. In fact, as the historian Gerald Grob has noted, supporters of the law believed it would provide the impetus for the elimination of "an institution that provided obsolete custodial care"—the hospital.[4] Such thinking reflected the new wave of studies in the social sciences that raised serious questions about the effectiveness of "total institutions" in treating persons with mental illness and particularly in preparing them to return to their communities.[5] As we have seen, popular suspicion of large institutions had been growing since World War II. Moreover, the focus on the community in the 1960s represented a logical outgrowth of the mental hygiene movement's founding principles. From its outset, the movement had sought to redirect attention, and resources, to the social and environmental rather than innate causes of mental illness—which it viewed as the key to explaining and treating the majority of individuals with mental illness. By the 1960s, the leading proponents of these views came from the ranks of a new subfield, community psychiatry, which called for the spread of services to all populations and whose members were more oriented toward social activism than their colleagues in clinical psychiatry. Influenced by the social and political movements of the day, community psychiatrists advocated for more mental health resources for disadvantaged urban communities and for a restructuring of services around geographical areas to provide comprehensive prevention and treatment. This viewpoint found support at the federal level in 1965 when the Johnson administration amended the law to include $73.5 million to support staffing of the new clinics.[6] Equally as important were amendments to the Social Security Act of 1935, which included psychiatric benefits for the elderly for the first time and thus contributed to a significant drop in the number of aged patients in state mental hospitals after 1965.[7] Taken together, these policy changes resulted in a drop in new admissions to state mental hospitals with a sharp increase in the use of outpatient clinics. In 1955 more than three-fourths of all "patient care episodes" occurred in hospitals and less than a quarter in outpatient clinics; by 1968 the respective numbers were 47.3 percent and 52.7 percent.[8]

In spite of the "anti-mental health movement" described in the previous chapter, Texas reformers found the state-level political climate to be supportive of these new opportunities. After 1962, the governor's mansion was occupied by John Connally, a Democrat who had served in Kennedy's administration and who had lent his support to the passage of the state's first mental health code in 1957. Almost immediately after the federal government authorized community mental health planning grants in 1963, Connally formed the Citizens Task Force for Community Mental Health to develop what became known as the Texas Plan for Mental Health. Helping to shape the work of the task force was a study conducted by the Hogg Foundation between 1958 and 1960 titled "Bridging the Gap." The study surveyed the reintegration experiences of patients released from state mental hospitals into their communities and highlighted the need for community-based services. This chapter begins with an examination of "Bridging the Gap," followed by a discussion of the Texas Plan, which was led by veterans of the mental health reform campaigns of the preceding decade, including virtually all the leadership of the Foundation. After an appraisal of the Texas Plan and the resulting creation of the TDMHMR, the chapter concludes with a discussion of an incident that dramatized the need for community-based services in a particular type of setting: the university campus. The incident was the notorious mass shooting that occurred at the University of Texas in 1966, which left twenty-three people dead, including the shooter, Charles Whitman. The Whitman episode underscored the need for preventive mental health services in the community generally and on college campuses in particular. Occurring in the Foundation's own proverbial backyard, it galvanized mental health reformers and illustrated just how much work remained to be done even after the landmark expansion of community mental health clinics and inauguration of the TDMHMR.

"Bridging the Gap"

For mental health reformers, the enactment of Texas' first mental health code in 1957 represented an important but preliminary step. "[A] prerequisite to the modernization of Texas laws relating to mental illness," as stated by the Texas Research League, the code set the stage for "the development of new laws which will enable mentally ill persons to be speedily admitted to treatment centers and rapidly discharged when cured." It was hoped that the code would help promulgate a new view of people with mental illness as individuals experiencing temporary conditions that could be "cured" in many cases with "early intensive treatment" in their communities, rather than individuals who were "invariably dangerous and in need of confinement."[9] Hoping to explore this thesis further, in the spring of 1958 the Hogg Foundation announced that it had been awarded a $50,000 grant from the National Institute of Mental Health to conduct "a two-year study on 'Bridging the Gap from Hospital to Community.'"[10] With director Sutherland serving as the principal investigator, the study focused on two state hospitals and four nearby communities, each with a population of less than 50,000. The goal was to examine the extent to which former patients were accepted back into their families and communities after being released from a state mental hospital. A team of researchers under Sutherland's supervision first surveyed the general population by having women's groups distribute the surveys. More in-depth surveys were conducted with selected opinion leaders about their attitudes toward mental illness, hospitalization, and hospitalized people. Finally, researchers identified and interviewed at least thirty former patients, as well as their families or nearest contacts, in each of the selected communities; ultimately, about 430 individual patient cases were reviewed. Occasionally the patient joined the family interview. Follow-up interviews were conducted approximately six months later. Initially, as he told the Texas Medical Association in garnering its cooperation, Sutherland hoped the project would result in a book that would illustrate the need for more community mental health services to help "rehabilitate" returned patients.[11] However, very early in the planning stages, Sutherland and his colleagues began to rethink the concept of "rehabilitation":

> What do we mean by rehabilitation? Dr. Sutherland commented we might even drop the word rehabilitation from our study. . . . Dr. Sutherland said that he felt this study might do well to shift off of attention to the patient as such and attend itself to the social structure in which the returned patient becomes a participant. Dr. Sutherland said we might also find to what extent a community can tolerate a-typical [sic] ways of contributing to the community by the former mental patient.[12]

As the locale for mental health reform shifted out of the institution into the community, the contexts of mental health and mental illness began to change. For the "Bridging the Gap" study, Sutherland suggested a focus on the community as well as the individual patient. This emphasis cut against the grain of the prevalent thinking of the 1950s, when "adjustment" had become a mantra for psychiatrists and psychologists attempting to explain all manner of behaviors from juvenile delinquency to the simmering discontent of suburban housewives. Moreover, by highlighting the community's role in accepting a former patient without reservations, Sutherland evoked his own sociological training and called for a more interdisciplinary— and less "medical"—approach to mental health and illness. What this meant in practice, for Sutherland, was that "adjustment" should be viewed as reciprocal with regard to people with mental illness. Importantly, however, the twenty-first-century phrase "people with mental illness," which implies a dynamic concept of mental illness, did not govern the thinking of mental health reformers in the 1950s and 1960s. Instead, they envisioned mental illness in the language of "cures" and "relapses"; discharged patients required community-based services and supportive attitudes from their families and communities to avoid a "relapse." Thus, the "Bridging the Gap" study explored the extent to which communities "adjusted" to discharged patients, offering them acceptance in reintegrating into their communities but within a mid-century framework.

Interviews with community members in the areas around Terrell State Hospital and the psychiatric unit at the University of Texas Medical Branch at Galveston suggested that discharged hospital patients rarely met with community acceptance. Field interviews in Paris and Snyder, Texas, produced comments from business owners stating that while they would "socialize" with former patients, they "wouldn't trust former patients in business dealings."[13] Clinical services also proved hard to come by, in part due to resistance from nearby general practitioners, who viewed such endeavors as redundant or even threatening to their own private practices. One physician respondent, who had considered specializing in psychiatry, noted that his colleagues were reluctant to refer patients to psychiatrists, preferring to offer informal counseling themselves. They would not "accept the fact that psychiatry is here to stay. . . . He [the physician] said education for mental health should start with the doctors—that is the group that we have got to reach somehow."[14] To their surprise, researchers found that some existing challenges had worsened as a result of the new mental health code. In Paris, the county judge was experiencing a growing number of requests from individuals who "came to talk to him about relatives with mental problems." In addition, "many people come in and ask to be committed themselves." The judge threw up his hands to the Foundation researchers, saying, "I can't help them, I don't know what to do," while looking to emulate a new counseling program offered in the courts of nearby Tyler.

Ironically, in Odessa, one of the hotbeds of anti-mental health feeling, researchers found one of the only communities where "a very positive, active organization developed whose objective it was to help the state hospital system improve their patient care and work with patients." A local "resistance group," tied to the region's anti-mental health movement, published a lengthy editorial in Odessa's local newspaper and managed to frustrate researchers' attempts to conduct a community survey.[15] These critics "were not anti-mental illness, they were anti-mental health," in that they welcomed discharged patients while opposing any organized expressions of mental health in the community. Thanks in part to an oil boom and a resulting high demand for laborers, researchers found, local citizens "really didn't care where the person came from, or who he was, as long as he could work and earn. Their emphasis upon these consummatory values made them relegate the condition of being an ex-patient to an unimportant factor."[16]

By 1960, having completed "extensive" interviews and surveys in several counties, researchers concluded that they had uncovered a "liberalization of attitudes" about mental illness, although these shifts suffered from an "action lag" in tangible supports for discharged patients.[17] Moreover, thanks to the mental health awareness campaigns of the preceding decade, which had utilized mass media, attitudes had improved similarly in both rural and urban areas.[18] Excerpts from the interviews themselves suggested a range of opinions as well as a lack of resources to assist discharged patients in transitioning into their respective communities.[19] There was "Cesspool Charlie," the sewage maintenance worker who "wore peculiar clothes and talked kinda funny"; he responded to teasing from local youths by displaying "his discharge paper from the state hospital" as proof that he was not "crazy." One businessman told researchers that he thought "ex-mental patients" could not be trusted, should not be employed, and in fact should be confined indefinitely in the hospitals: "we haven't got any place for them here." Other informants lamented the lack of community resources. "Our hands are tied," stated a social worker. "All of our assistance is done in terms of $2.00 or $5.00, and the problems that these people have are so much greater that we just can't do anything about it . . . it hurts." However, some interviewees praised the state hospitals for helping loved ones who could not remain in the community. One man described the family's trepidation at the prospect of transferring his mother from an "expensive" private facility to the state hospital, "because we knew what an awful place it was." In the end, the family ended up "amazed" at the quality of the facility and the staff, extolling the hospital as "the best treatment center in Texas, public or private." While these anecdotes were short on key details, they presented a decidedly mixed impression that illustrated some progress in viewpoints about mental illness and services provided to people with mental illness.

Of equal concern to researchers were differences in attitudes toward mental health and mental illness along racial and ethnic lines. Among the publications emerging from the research was a study that contrasted white and African American views of mental illness. Researchers concluded that racial discrimination had left African Americans somewhat cut off from the public discourse on mental health. Moreover, community-based services were not available to them; in a case of perceived mental illness, the only available option was a state mental hospital. As a result, the commitment rate was much higher for African Americans than for whites, and black male patients had the lowest possibility of release of any category of patients in the state mental hospitals. However, researchers discovered that black patients found greater acceptance (though no greater resources) upon their return to the community.[20] Meanwhile, an internal report profiled a twenty-eight-year-old "Latin" patient who became frustrated by workplace discrimination; he was a construction worker who was prevented from advancing into a skilled trade and was told by his white supervisor that "he was asking for something he shouldn't." The report concluded that discrimination may have contributed to a diagnosis of mental illness in this individual's case.[21]

"Bridging the Gap" resulted in a few journal publications and a series of public lectures but not the book-length study originally envisioned by Sutherland. However, the study suggested the limits of old-line mental hospitals. Even when they performed reasonably well, large institutions carried an enduring social stigma that inhibited the ability of people with mental illness to find acceptance in their communities. Moreover, mental health reformers increasingly became convinced that the vast majority of people with mental illness could receive effective treatment in community rather than institutional settings. While they long had advocated for the development of "outpatient clinics," as we have seen, mental health reformers by the early 1960s began to assert the notion that a comprehensive system of such clinics could not only supplement large institutions but possibly replace them outright. The Hogg Foundation arrived at this conclusion shortly before the publication of *Action for Mental Health* and thus welcomed the report's call for "the eventual abolition of the large state mental hospital as we know it today in favor of smaller, intensive treatment units, integrated with other agencies and facilities at the community level." In reviewing the report for the *Journal of Clinical Psychology*, psychology professor and Hogg Foundation associate Ira Iscoe pointedly asked whether "clinical psychology [will] support such a radical yet progressive step, or are we already too institutionalized in our own approaches to diagnosis and treatment?"[22] By the time it appeared in print, Iscoe's challenge was being taken up by a task force charged with developing a statewide plan for mental health services.

"Trying to Catch Up With the Twentieth Century": The Texas Plan for Mental Health

In addition to the impetus provided by the publication of *Action for Mental Health* in 1961, the annual National Governor's Conference adopted a resolution at its 1962 meeting for each state to develop a "comprehensive master plan" for mental health services.[23] In anticipation of the federal Community Mental Health Centers Act, the Texas State Department of Health formed the Office of Mental Health Planning in February 1963. This office supported a four-person executive committee, chaired by James E. Peavy, the commissioner of health. The other committee members included Cyril J. Ruilmann, the director of Mental Health and Hospitals for the BTSHSS; C.L. Abernathy, a judge from Plainview in northern Texas who had been active in mental health issues; and Robert L. Sutherland, executive director of the Hogg Foundation.[24] The committee's work in the initial year was funded by a grant from the National Institute for Mental Health of $180,000 for 1963–64.[25] The first issue before the committee was whether to pursue federal funds at all; the influential Texas Medical Association voiced opposition to accepting funds even though it expressed support for mental health, seemingly on the basis of a more generalized and oft-stated antipathy to "socialized medicine." This position represented a departure from its parent organization, the American Medical Association, which the previous fall had sponsored the First National Congress on Mental Illness and Health and articulated a set of recommendations supporting the creation of a system of community mental health clinics.[26] The committee overruled this objection, arguing that the planning grant sought "to aid the states in working out their own problems rather than imposing some type of federal control on the operation of program."[27] In May 1963, the executive committee submitted its first application for federal funds under the new program. The proposal called for a seventeen-member steering committee and a massive citizens committee comprising more than one hundred individuals from a variety of backgrounds, including the mental health professions, elected officials, and prominent private citizens. In July 1963, the committee received its first allotment of a two-year planning grant totaling roughly $370,000 under the new federal law.[28]

The committee met several times during the summer, articulating the goals for the Texas Plan for Mental Health, mapping out further the structure of the citizens committee that would develop the plan, and identifying and responding to challenges to the implementation of expanded community mental health services.[29] In October 1963, the committee issued a short written statement titled "The Future Is Now: Statewide and Community Planning for Mental Health Services."[30] Striking a pragmatic tone, the document called for "broad participation of the professional citizens and governmental leaders of the state in the formulation of this comprehensive plan" to ensure "that these leaders will assume responsibility for its effective implementation."[31] Such broad participation was recommended by the National Institute of Mental Health as a guideline for grant applicants, reflecting a belief that involvement in the planning process would inculcate a sense of ownership in the outcome of the reform enterprise. "Enormous efforts have been made in the past in Texas in planning for mental health," the report noted, "but the fact that they have not been fully implemented may reflect the fact that citizen leadership was not systematically involved in either the planning or its implementation." The ambitious statement of goals called for a plan "to preserve, protect, and promote the mental health of all Texans" by making available preventive care, diagnosis, treatment, and rehabilitative services in communities rather than only in institutional settings. Seeking to reassure physicians, the document included a section titled "What the Plan Means to the Medical Profession," which recited the American Medical Association's endorsement of "multiple source financing for community mental health services" and "the need for additional expenditures at all levels."[32] In response, the Texas Medical Association adopted a resolution urging its members "to cooperate in this comprehensive mental health planning effort." The resolution singled out private practitioners, asking them to provide aggregated data on patients "whose primary problem is of mental mal-functioning."[33]

One week before the committee issued "The Future Is Now," Governor Connally delivered a keynote address to the annual meeting of the Texas Association for Mental Health in Dallas. "We are standing on the threshold of important new progress," he began, "in our campaign to solve this most urgent of all health problems."[34] Connally identified three major goals: prevention; "early, uninterrupted treatment and care close to the patient's home"; and positive mental health, which he described as "helping people strengthen the 'emotional muscle' needed to overcome daily problems and occasional major crises." In elaborating on prevention, Connally provided a powerful illustration that also pushed back against the objections of some segments of the medical profession:

> On the first point of prevention, we understand about preventive medicine. We accept on faith and without thought the protection of our physical well-being by the medical profession. We have faith that the water we drink is pure. We have faith that the food we eat is free of harmful bacteria. . . . When we look at the mental illnesses, however, we are told by our medical scientists that much too little is known to develop an adequate preventive program. The word "prevention" defies precise definition when applied to the mental illnesses. As in so many areas, we already know much better than we do. There is ample medical and scientific evidence that early identification of mental illness, early and intensive treatment, and easily available after-care will hold to a minimum the seriously disabling effects. Of the nearly 5,000 Texans who voluntarily entered a state mental hospital last year, how many might have been able to remain at home, perhaps continuing to earn a living and to take care of their families, if they had found the help they sought—months or even years earlier?[35]

Although Connally praised the "remarkable changes" in the state's mental hospitals, he made it clear that most people in need of mental health services could receive them where they "lived and worked" and "not in a hospital 300 miles away after a trying commitment procedure." Only a small number of people with mental illness, he suggested, required the "intensive treatment" of a mental hospital. The state now operated nine mental health clinics, up from four during the 1950s, which served about four thousand patients during the previous year. More clinics were needed, however, for children as well as adults. In addition, more training was needed for the "family physicians, clergymen, teachers, and social and welfare agencies who most often see mental or emotional disability in its early stages." Addressing all of these goals required "cooperation" and "coordination" across a range of agencies, a challenge that Connally characterized as an "obligation" for mental health reformers. While he did not specify any particular solution or advocate for the creation a dedicated state agency, Connally nevertheless conveyed a sense of unprecedented possibility.

The group charged with realizing that potential was the General Planning Committee, also known as the Statewide Citizens' Committee on Mental Health Program Planning, a 116-member body that began meeting in January 1964. Included in this group were psychiatrists, psychologists, social workers, pediatricians, teachers, ministers, and private citizens who had been involved in mental health reform in some way. Wayne Holtzman, Bernice Milburn Moore, and Bert Kruger Smith of the Hogg Foundation served on this committee. The committee's composition was overwhelmingly white and male, with only a handful of women and one African American and Latino member.[36] This larger committee was chaired by Abernathy and co-chaired by Sutherland. Together with a "psychiatrist-coordinator," Abernathy and Sutherland organized this huge group into thirteen separate task forces: Legislative, Public Education, Prevention, Services to Troubled People, Diagnosis and Treatment—Children, Diagnosis and Treatment—Adults, Rehabilitation, Finance, Epidemiology, Research, Training and Recruitment, Facilities and Construction, and Administration and Coordination. The fundamental question confronting this committee was stated by the psychiatrist-coordinator during a conference with consultant Archie Foley, a faculty member in the Division of Community Psychiatry at Columbia University's School of Public Health: "What should we be aspiring toward if we are trying to catch up with the twentieth century and provide the kind of community mental health services that are alleged to be desirable?"[37] Foley argued for a focus on promoting mental health rather than responding to mental illness, which in turn required not only providing clinical services but also empowering "the first line of defense people . . . the caretakers who come in contact with people who may be developing psychological disorders . . . teachers, ministers, probation officers, the court."[38]

Over the course of the year, the committee gathered a significant amount of information. It surveyed all the social service organizations it could locate around the state, gathered salary data for mental health professionals working in public agencies, compared mental health research grant dollars in Texas against California and national averages, collected the educational backgrounds of mental health and related professionals, and tabulated the mental health treatment resources in the major and mid-level population centers of Texas.[39] The results showed that Texas lagged far behind other states in many of these categories. Salaries of psychiatric social workers, chief psychologists, and staff psychologists ranked well behind the eight other most comparable states by population. Only one-fifth of all employed social workers in Texas held appropriate educational credentials in social work. Students who earned medical degrees in psychiatry in Texas typically left the state to find higher paying employment elsewhere; "Texas is training psychiatrists for other states," concluded the Task Force on Training and Recruitment. "We train them and they move to Louisiana or Kansas or some other place."[40] Perhaps the most revealing data set was a survey of mental health treatment resources in the state's twenty-one largest population centers. Unsurprisingly, the Dallas–Fort Worth, Houston–Galveston, and Austin–San Antonio regions led in the number of professionals, hospital beds, and clinical services. However, the disparity with the remaining regions was stark, with several of them lacking any clinical services and some employing fewer than five mental health professionals. Notably, Laredo, the largest population center in the Rio Grande Valley, employed no professionals and offered no clinical or hospital services of any kind.[41]

These disparities in service levels led the committee to one of its core recommendations, for a central statewide agency to administer mental health services. A survey of mental health providers also returned numerous responses calling for such an agency, even as they acknowledged the likely opposition of conservative activists suspicious of government intervention. One response, sent to the Services to Troubled People Task Force, labeled such concerns "a symptom of social pathology" and went on as follows:

> Persons who look at government as "them" as opposed to private or voluntary efforts as "us" disclose their lack of faith in democracy and tend to increase rather than decrease this dangerous and needless dichotomy. A central mental health authority should be . . . guided by the philosophy that while the least amount of government might be best, the fact remains that government of the people governs the best and the emphasis should be on quality of government not quantity.[42]

The final report of the committee, titled *The Texas Plan for Mental Health Services*, was completed on December 1, 1964. The 250-page report included thirteen sections with the findings and recommendations of each of the task forces created under the General Planning Committee. However, two core recommendations stood out: the creation of "a single mental health authority—the Texas Department of Mental Health," to replace the disparate agencies and subagencies handling different aspects of mental health services, and the establishment of "comprehensive mental health centers . . . in at least 21 metropolitan centers." The Texas Plan thus called for a sweeping administrative reorganization that, in its view, would combine the functions of the BTSHSS and the Division of Mental Health within the Department of Health, both units that had been created in the preceding two decades. In addition, while the plan did recommend some improvements to the state hospitals and special schools, it clearly envisioned a reduction in their use with a corresponding increase in the use of community mental health centers. Indeed, most of the second-tier recommendations derived from the anticipated expansion of these centers. For example, the report suggested locating centers near medical schools wherever possible to support research and training, as well as developing facilities especially for children's mental health, expanding counseling services in public schools, and providing specialized services for the elderly.[43]

At least one of the committee's leaders felt uncertain about the likely reception of the Texas Plan. In August 1964, the psychiatrist-coordinator Moody Bettis of Houston had suggested extending the planning process into the next year, but Sutherland prodded him to present the committee's major findings and recommendations to Governor Connally sooner rather than later. "Move more rapidly and have firm recommendations ready for this coming Legislature," he advised, to build on public interest rather than "delay a presentation of a state plan until two years from now," when "much of the momentum will be lost."[44] Three days after the report was sent to Governor Connally, Bettis circulated a memo to the General Planning Committee urging members to "help put it over" by talking with their legislators, county judges, city mayors, local newspapers, and civic clubs over the next six months, "spanning the 59th regular session of the Texas Legislature."[45]

The Texas Plan had received generally favorable press coverage throughout the planning process. A spate of articles highlighted long-standing issues of low per-patient state spending in the mental hospitals, with Texas ranking near the bottom among the states.[46] Special impetus seemed to arise from the Kennedy assassination. A committee spokesperson told the *Austin Statesman* that the assassination made it "dreadfully apparent" that "we are years late in mental health planning," noting that "[Lee Harvey] Oswald had a history of mental illness as a young man, but referrals to health agencies were not followed through."[47] The committee's Public Relations Task Force wrote and disseminated press releases at strategic times in the planning process, focusing attention particularly on data illustrating the lack of community services around the state.[48] One measure of the effectiveness of this approach was the lack of controversy attending the release of the Texas Plan and the subsequent legislative process during the spring 1965 session. The only significant change made during the legislative process was the addition of mental retardation services, reflecting a similar emphasis at the national level as well as the growing influence of advocacy groups for individuals with intellectual and developmental disabilities. The Texas Association for Retarded Children, as well as a separate state task force on mental retardation, had arrived at similar conclusions regarding the formation of a statewide agency and the establishment of community-based services. When the legislature combined the recommendations of the two task forces into a single bill, these groups threw their support behind it.[49] Otherwise, House Bill 3, the Texas Mental Health and Mental Retardation Act, passed through both houses of the legislature and was signed into law by Governor Connally on April 5, 1965. Media reports focused largely on the law's call for community mental health centers. The *Houston Post* reported that the law would "entail a shift over the next 10 years from institutional care in state mental hospitals and special schools to 'community care,' in or near the affected person's home," while the *Austin Statesman* noted that city and county governments would need to increase their spending on mental health and mental retardation services.[50]

The new law abolished the BTSHSS and the Division of Mental Health within the Texas State Department of Health, combining their functions under a new agency, the TDMHMR. An appointed nine-person board of directors governed the TDMHMR, which appointed a commissioner, who in turn supervised two deputy commissioners, respectively, for mental health and mental retardation. The agency thus assumed responsibility for the state hospitals and special schools, as well as community centers that would be constructed around the state. The TDMHMR grew rapidly over the subsequent decades to become the largest state agency in Texas. By the early 1990s, the TDMHMR was operating sixty-two facilities, including hospitals, community mental health and mental retardation centers, and various specialized treatment facilities. The TDMHMR also oversaw county, city, and regional mental health and mental retardation agencies, which in turn established a range of group homes, transitional facilities, vocational rehabilitation services, and case management services.[51]

The advent of the TDMHMR represented a watershed moment not only for the state of Texas but also for the Hogg Foundation for Mental Health. For over two decades, the Foundation had worked toward the establishment of policies and allocation of resources that would foment "positive mental health" and support more humane treatment of people with mental illness. To a great extent, it appeared that goal had been realized. Although it would continue to award planning grants to the TDMHMR, after 1965 the Foundation began to withdraw from direct involvement in the public policy arena and the issues surrounding institutional and clinical treatment of mental illness, leaving those fields to the TDMHMR; the growing number of university departments of psychiatry, psychology, and social work emerging around the state; and the professional and advocacy organizations related to mental health and mental retardation.[52] Even amid its involvement with the development of the TDMHMR, the Foundation had been active in other areas, particularly two burgeoning fields of activity in the 1960s: campus mental health and community action demonstration programs.

A "Cycle of Recurring Tragedies": Community Action and Mental Health

The culmination of the Texas Plan coincided with a shifting focus at the Hogg Foundation on community-based demonstration programs in mental health. In 1965 the Foundation announced a new emphasis on the "encouragement and testing of new patterns in mental health education and community action; early detection and prevention of emotional difficulties; and treatment and rehabilitation."[53] These goals would be supported through an expanded grants-in-aid program "made to departments and branches of the University, to community agencies, and to state-wide organizations . . . to demonstrate and evaluate new patterns of work in the above areas."[54] For her part, Ima Hogg, while pleased with the Foundation's leadership role in major public policy reforms, felt that the Foundation had become sufficiently influential by the late 1950s to mount a "sustained and successful plan of action" as "an example for other communities to follow."[55] Both Hogg and Sutherland were enamored with the model being put forward by the Ford Foundation's "grey areas" program, which provided grant funds to demonstration projects in inner-city areas, and subsequently by President Kennedy's Committee on Juvenile Delinquency and Youth Crime, formed in 1961. Soon after Ima expressed these views to Sutherland, he was appointed to the review committees for both organizations, which together represented a new model for responding to newly discovered poverty, particularly in inner-city areas. The model called for the identification of a "demonstration area," typically a specific neighborhood or set of neighborhoods defined by demographic, economic, and other statistical factors, and the identification and development of needed services in collaboration with community leaders selected by local residents. An early example of this "community action" model could be found in Mobilization for Youth, which began in New York City under the leadership of child psychologist Kenneth Clark in 1959 with funding from the Ford Foundation. Similar antidelinquency and antipoverty programs surfaced in large and mid-sized cities around the nation during the 1960s, funded later under the Office of Economic Opportunity as part of President Lyndon Johnson's War on Poverty.

In July 1963, the Ford Foundation awarded the Hogg Foundation a five-year grant for a project titled "Philanthropy in the Southwest." Under the terms of this grant, matching funds would be provided for community action demonstration projects in mental health and social services with an evaluation component.[56] That same year, the President's Committee made one of its first awards under its community action program to Houston Action for Youth, an anti-delinquency program that ran for three years. Led by the psychology department at the University of Houston and the Houston Community Council, Houston Action for Youth organized several youth service programs, some of which were taken over by Head Start, Job Corps, and other agencies after the grant expired.[57] In 1968 the Foundation funded the Juvenile Law Policy Project, which was housed in the University of Texas Law School's Southwest Center for Law and the Behavioral Sciences, itself a multiyear project designed and executed with significant Foundation input.[58] The project's director, law professor Robert O. Dawson, later would recall that the Foundation provided important support for the project's rewriting of Texas' juvenile and family codes over a period of several years.[59] After a federal lawsuit resulted in an overhaul of the state's juvenile justice system, Dawson began to work with the Foundation on reform of the juvenile training schools.[60]

Many of the projects funded by the Hogg Foundation, usually in collaboration with one of the private or public agencies on whose boards Robert Sutherland served, embraced the "community action" model. An indicative project was the Clayton Homes Neighborhood Development Program, begun in 1959 by the Neighborhood Centers Association of Houston and Harris County (NCA). An umbrella organization of the area's historic settlement houses and community centers, the NCA operated largely in Houston's poorest neighborhoods. In 1961 NCA director Franklin Harbach, a social worker from New York who moved to Houston during World War II, began corresponding with Robert Sutherland about acquiring grant funds for the Clayton Homes project. The NCA had set up intensive child care, youth recreation, parent education, vocational training, and clinical mental health services in the housing project, which had been built in 1952 in the largely Mexican American Second Ward. These programs were developed under the shared governance of social workers and local residents on the Clayton Homes Neighborhood Development Program Committee. With financial assistance from the NCA, the Clayton Homes committee opened a locally owned grocery store; enrolled children in pre-K, kindergarten, and elementary school; and sponsored adults who wished to take night classes at the local high school.[61] With Sutherland's guidance and support, the NCA received funding from the National Institutes of Health and the Ford Foundation supporting the Clayton Homes demonstration project. Notably, the proposal described the Clayton Homes program in the language of community mental health. "Our experience to date," it stated, "indicates that individuals and families . . . experience growth and development as they plan and work together in self-help neighborhood development projects such as beautification, school bus transportation, or neighborhood traffic control." The demonstration program focused especially on "promoting positive and preventive mental health on the neighborhood level," with the ultimate goal of fostering a "therapeutic neighborhood," a term adapted from the "therapeutic community" theorized by community psychiatrists of the period (see chapter 3).[62] So successful was the Clayton Homes project by 1963 that NCA director Harbach highlighted the project's "mental health implications for urban areas" in talks given to the Boston Settlement Council and the National Institute of Mental Health and responded to numerous inquiries about the model.[63]

Even amid this flurry of activity, concern continued to grow with regard to the perception of continually lagging levels of preventive mental health services. In a 1959 letter, Miss Ima had envisioned "a cycle of recurring tragedies" followed by "calls for remedies, expert opinions, and recommendations, and then nothing happens," usually due to a lack of funds.[64] Around the same time, University of Texas president Harry Ransom wrote to Sutherland about the lack of attention given to mental health issues on the campus. He wrote,

> On the American campus, I encounter constant problems in "mental health" which seem to be the concern of nobody . . . But so far as I can see, there is no concerted effort to look at the state University as a community potentially unhealthy in its condition of mind. I mean this quite seriously. Our forefathers gave lip service—often in ancient tongues—to ideals like *mens sana in corpore sano* (a sound mind in a sound body); but neither they nor we have ever confronted the problem of establishing bases of judgment for the mental health of the state University.[65]

These warnings appeared prescient in the wake of the violent events that took place in Texas in the 1960s. Immediately after the Kennedy assassination, the Foundation funded an attitude survey of two hundred Dallas residents. Writing about the study to a colleague, Sutherland lamented the "numerous trends" that, in his view, had contributed to the tragedy. "Did you know," he wrote, "that Oswald was picked up on a delinquency charge at the age of 13 in New York and after psychological examination, he was thought to have definite schizophrenic tendencies, to be dangerous, and that he should be committed. The court did not follow the advice of the examiner."[66]

For many observers, a painful validation of these concerns arose from the mass shooting carried out on the University of Texas campus by Charles Whitman on August 1, 1966. A former Marine and engineering student, Whitman killed his mother and his wife on the morning of August 1 before making his way to the top of the iconic tower, where administration offices and the Hogg Foundation's own offices were housed, around 11:30 that morning. After he reached the twenty-seventh floor, Whitman bludgeoned and killed a receptionist, shot several other onlookers, and climbed the remaining two floors to the observation deck, armed with six guns, knives, and other supplies. He subsequently opened fire on persons walking around the university campus as well as nearby streets, killing ten and wounding thirty-one before police were able to make their way to the observation deck, where an exchange of fire resulted in Whitman's death. The Hogg Foundation's offices were located on the twenty-fourth floor of the Tower, five flights below the observation deck where Whitman stood for approximately ninety minutes firing at random individuals. About a dozen Foundation staff members were present that day, and their recollections were published by the Foundation in pamphlets and press releases. They reported hearing Whitman's shots that killed the first victims on the observation deck; barricading themselves in their offices as they heard the "fusillade" of bullets rain down on passersby on campus and nearby Guadalupe Street; hearing screams and seeing victims felled, many of whom were known to Foundation staff, and being unable to assist them; and frantically calling colleagues and loved ones. Casualties included a recent high school graduate who had given swimming lessons to Robert Sutherland's grandson, killed along with his girlfriend while they stood in front of the campus bookstore, and a graduate student who had been a houseguest of Wayne Holtzman, shot while walking along Guadalupe Street, leaving behind a wife and five children. "It was truly a nightmare at noon," recalled one staff member. "Campus mental health never seemed more important."[67]

Governor Connally concurred with that sentiment, taking emergency steps after the incident. He charged an eleven-member committee, comprised of prominent psychiatrists and medical professionals from around the nation and chaired by Foundation director Sutherland, with investigating the reasons why an ostensibly upright citizen and ex-Marine had engaged in mass murder and with recommending actions that could be taken to prevent future tragedies. The investigation uncovered a history of personal and family problems beneath the seemingly friendly façade that Whitman had presented to many of his fellow students. About four months before the Tower shooting, in late March 1966, Whitman had visited the university health center, where he met with staff psychiatrist Maurice D. Heatly, who talked with him for about an hour. Heatly's notes from the session described Whitman's distress over his parents' ongoing separation; his mother had left his father and moved from the family's home in Florida to stay with her son in Austin. Whitman also had experienced his own marital troubles, along with a history of violent outbursts. His greatest frustration, however, stemmed from feelings of failure; Whitman desperately wanted to surpass his father's achievements yet worried that he had fallen behind his own peers, many of whom had finished college and embarked on careers. As an illustration of his sometimes violent fantasies, during the health center session Whitman had described a vision of "going up on the Tower with a deer rifle and shooting people." Heatly did not believe Whitman was serious, however, because students often used the Tower as a prop for such statements without acting on them. Heatly's notes described Whitman as "an all-American boy" whose troubles could be managed through a series of one-on-one sessions. He dismissed Whitman with a recommendation to schedule a future appointment, which Whitman did not keep.[68] Like many others who had known Whitman, the psychiatrist had not believed him capable of mass violence. "The whole thing is an enigma," psychiatry professor and Foundation consultant Ira Iscoe later told the *Houston Chronicle*. "It would be easier to understand if he had been one of the campus Beatniks, bearded, unkempt, and on scholastic probation, aimlessly protesting a variety of things and meandering along with no purpose in life . . . look at Whitman—clean, neat, crew cut, good grades and a purpose in life." Wayne Holtzman, who had witnessed the shooting from his corner office in Sutton Hall directly across from the Tower, told reporters that early identification of such cases was difficult "even with a fully staffed counseling center."[69]

The committee examined every facet of Whitman's personal history, interviewing numerous individuals who had known him throughout his life and reviewing medical and educational documents dating back to his early childhood. An autopsy would later uncover that Whitman had been taking Dexedrine, an amphetamine, although it could not determine for certain if the drug had been in his system on the day of the shooting (Whitman's body was embalmed before the autopsy) and the existence of a brain tumor, which may have contributed to extreme mood swings including bouts of violent anger. However, the committee viewed these medical results as inconclusive and did not cite them as causes for Whitman's actions. Instead, its report cited his "profound personal dissatisfaction" and the range of personal and family problems as precipitating factors. Ultimately, the committee concluded that it could not state definitively what had caused Charles Whitman to commit mass murder, because he had not received a full psychiatric evaluation at any time prior to the Tower shooting.[70]

Although individual committee members may have concurred with Iscoe and Holtzman about the impossibility of definitively spotting a would-be Whitman, it nevertheless found itself on more solid footing with regard to its other charge to recommend prevention measures. The topic already had drawn attention due to social and cultural changes in the 1960s, as well as Sutherland's own professional experiences with campus mental health. He had worked at the University of Texas for twenty-five years; moreover, in the 1930s, prior to directing the Foundation, he had served as dean of students at Bucknell University. The year before the Tower shooting, the Foundation's national advisory council had included campus mental health in its wide-ranging discussions of emerging areas of need in the implementation of the federal and state mental health laws. Sutherland had characterized campus mental health as an "urgent and timely" topic due to the rapid growth of American public universities in the postwar era; increased research requirements for faculty members, which pulled them away from students; "growing restlessness and intellectual foment among students"; and the lack of qualified counselors.[71] Little was done, however, until a few months before the Whitman incident, when a request from the Board of Regents had promulgated the creation of a task force, chaired by Sutherland and including Iscoe, to recommend improvements to the university's student counseling services. The regent who had initiated the task force, Rabbi Levi Olan, was a forceful proponent of racial equality and public education who led one of the largest Jewish congregations in the nation in Dallas. Olan convened the task force in April 1966 with the goal of finding "a program which will meet students where they are, which will be suitable for all students—not just those in trouble. We should not insist that a student has to be in difficulty to qualify for attention."[72] At subsequent meetings, members complained that the university health center merged testing and counseling functions in the same department, with the result of minimizing resources to counseling. Student health services, they felt, "did not begin to meet the needs of students" and was "too psychiatrically oriented"; students had been heard saying that "you had to be some sort of nut" to visit counseling services. They also felt that faculty and staff members should be educated about mental health so that they could identify students who needed assistance; however, "the university culture" discouraged "the spending of time with students." As one member put it, "no built-in rewards for counseling" existed for faculty or staff.[73] At a July 20 meeting, less than two weeks before the Tower shooting, the task force identified a range of services that would fall under the rubric of "counseling," to include such features as academic advising, in-dormitory counseling services, an expanded new student orientation, religious counseling services, and peer group therapy sessions.[74] "I would like to focus on innovations in the provision of psychological services to students," wrote Ira Iscoe after the meeting, "[so that] it is possible for a student to go through a healthy identity crisis without being labeled emotionally disturbed or psychiatric."[75]

The Tower shooting understandably lent a new urgency to this project, as the task force's work essentially merged with that of the committee formed by Governor Connally. Although Sutherland chaired both committees, the driving force behind the push for more robust student counseling services came from Ira Iscoe. Originally from New York and Canada, Iscoe studied psychology at the University of California–Los Angeles (UCLA) under Roy Dorcus, a prominent figure in the field of clinical psychology. Iscoe joined the psychology faculty at the University of Texas in 1951; both he and his wife Louise Iscoe worked with the Hogg Foundation for the next several decades. The couple were vocal supporters of racial integration at the University of Texas; Ira recruited and taught some of the first African American students in the psychology program, while Louise authored a book, titled *Overcoming*, about the struggle to integrate the university in the 1950s and 1960s.[76] An early proponent of community mental health, Ira Iscoe had been closely involved behind the scenes in the campaign to reform the state hospitals and special schools, often by sending his students and graduates to work in the facilities. Iscoe would go on to direct student counseling at the university in its first decade of existence after the Tower shooting and founded the community psychology program in the 1970s, which trained an entire generation of psychologists.[77]

A few weeks after the Tower shooting, Iscoe went on a fact-finding trip to his alma mater, UCLA, to view its student counseling center, which was a stand-alone facility with an independent budget. He found that UCLA dedicated significantly more budgetary resources, including full-time staff positions in functions that were supported part-time at the University of Texas student health center. Many of the professional staff members at the Texas center held joint appointments with academic departments; by contrast, at UCLA Iscoe found that the staff were "devoted full-time to helping people." He also noted the "high level reception skills" even in the UCLA front-desk staff, allowing them to make appropriate intake and referral decisions to "the full range" of university services within and beyond the counseling center and the extensive use of "non-faculty personnel" at the center.[78] Iscoe singled out UCLA's intake counselor program for particular attention as a new innovation. Rather than assign each student walk-in or appointment for a regular fifty-minute counseling session days or even weeks in the future, the intake counselor assessed each student briefly in a discussion that could last as long as twenty minutes. According to Iscoe, this practice allowed for clearer assess-

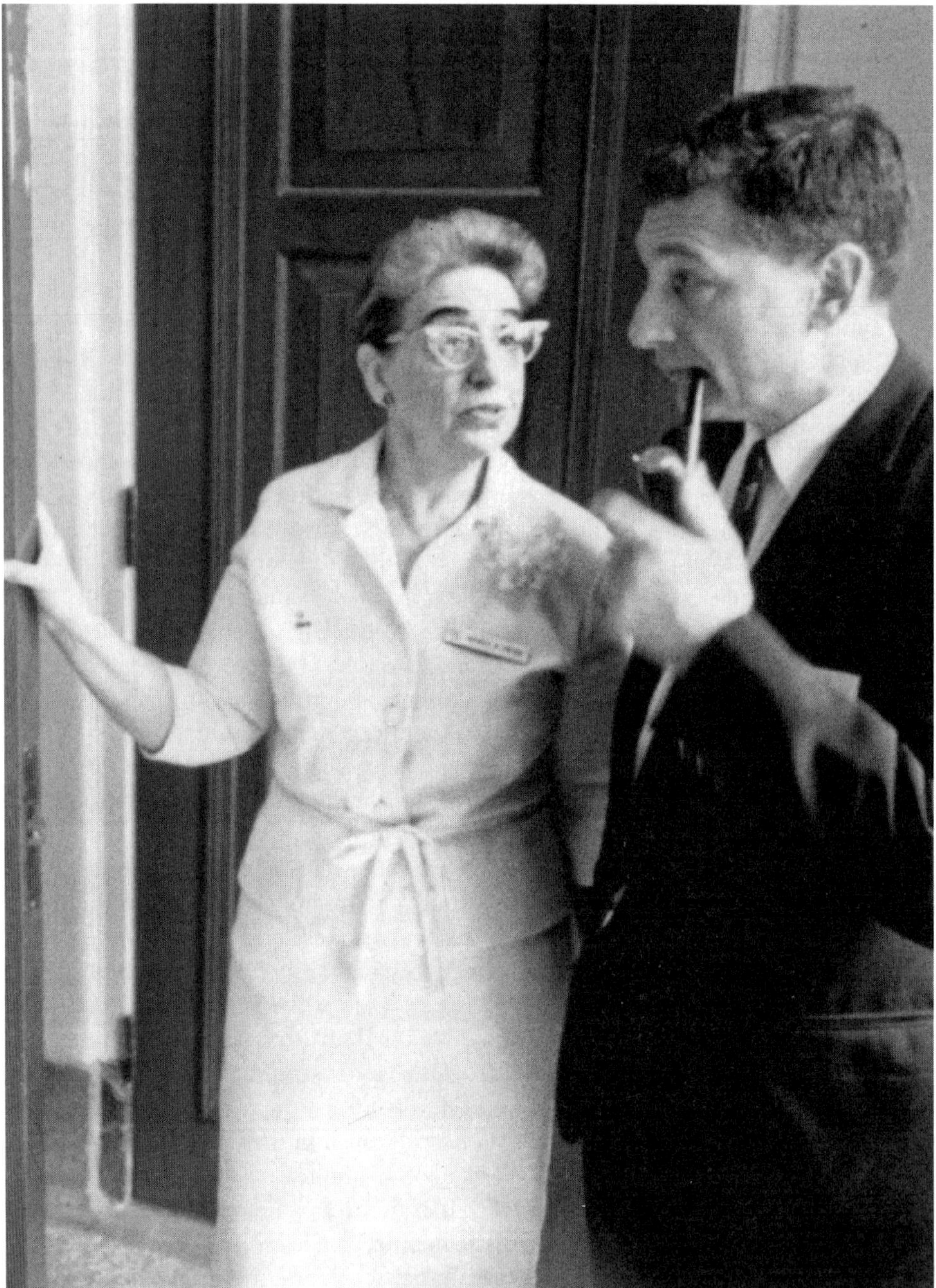

5.1. Bernice Milburn Moore and Ira Iscoe at the dedication of the Hogg Building, University of Texas at Austin, 1968, Box 98–285–15, Hogg Foundation Papers.

ment of emergency cases that needed immediate attention and also allowed the student to feel heard and thus be more likely to return for a scheduled appointment—an outcome that seemed especially relevant in light of Charles Whitman's experience at the University of Texas' student health center. With an overall enrollment of 25,000 students, UCLA had made "stringent efforts to reduce the impersonality of the school" (in the margin next to this statement appears Sutherland's handwritten note "alienation").[79]

Iscoe's report from UCLA decisively influenced the task force's approach. Should counseling on a college campus focus on a student's educational or emotional needs? Even "superior" students dropped out due to "adjustment" issues at a large, seemingly impersonal university. Sutherland summarized the problem against the historical sweep of mental health reform:

> As psychiatry came of age nationally, it also entered the college scene. To begin with, the psychiatric specialist saw students only on referral from other doctors in the health service or from deans. He treated students with major problems of emotional disturbance and of deviant social behavior. Later on, more students in the general range of "the normal" sought counseling on emotional problems. In many universities . . . the psychiatrist developed functions seemingly as much educational as medical. Such a point of view stressed preventive consultation with students and staff—a far broader approach than that of picking up the pieces after breakdown.[80]

The task force's preliminary recommendations, made in early September 1966, called for the development of "a broad health program for students and faculty," a "mental health program for students and faculty" that would serve as "a fitting memorial" to the victims of the Tower shooting, and the "development of an effective student counseling service" that was "personalized" and available to "each student in need at any time."[81] The recommendations were received favorably by academic administrators; in March 1967, Chancellor Harry Ransom presented them to the Board of Regents. "Because of both national and local conditions," the improvement of "systems of counseling in both general institutions and the medical schools" was "essential."[82] When confronted with resistance from the dean of students, who oversaw the university health center, the task force enlisted an important ally in the implementation process: students. In March 1967, Sutherland and Iscoe met with a group of students affiliated with the campus chapters of the YMCA and YWCA, who were functioning as informal counselors in their dormitories but who felt they lacked the appropriate training. These students "spoke unfavorably about the reception a student gets at Testing and Counseling," contrasting the impersonality of the center with the "people oriented" experience at the University of California at Berkeley, which they had visited. Sutherland coached the students on the best way to bypass the dean of students and approach the vice chancellor and chancellor with their concerns.[83] The combined pressure of Sutherland's task force and student groups, against the backdrop of the Tower shooting and the general perception of growing campus unrest, broke down any remaining resistance to the expansion of student counseling services. By the end of the 1967 spring semester, the university had begun implementation, including the separation of the testing and counseling centers into distinct units, each with a director; an increase in the number of full-time counselors at the health center; the hiring of graduate student counselors for undergraduate dormitories; and the development of a twenty-four-hour crisis hotline.[84] Begun in July 1967, the telephone hotline fielded more than 10,000 student calls during the first academic year of operation.[85] The service continued to grow over the next decade, under Iscoe's direction, from a "traditional ed psych service" focused on career advising into a comprehensive counseling service that "met students where they were":

> Before telephone counseling, you had sort of traditional, "don't bother us on Saturday afternoon," you know. The important thing was to involve faculty in the dormitories, the leaders . . . and most important, to have 24-hour telephone service. It made a huge difference. So whatever the excuse for the call, it's "I want to talk to somebody." And the other thing was that you had . . . laypeople, who had lived life but didn't have degrees in the field both answering the phone and in the counseling center who you gave some training to. They were not professional anybody. But they could listen.[86]

Iscoe quickly discovered that even the twenty-four-hour telephone hotline left some room for improvement, particularly because of its close association with counseling and mental illness. In response, he partnered with a local coffee shop, the Methodist student center, and the Austin-Travis County Mental Health Association to develop The Listening Ear.[87] Operating during after-hours and overnight hours only, The Listening Ear offered "listening" services in a nonclinical setting with coffee, tea, and pastries. It pointedly described itself as "*not* a counseling center but rather a place where a person can share his frustrations, anxieties or fears and hopefully, thereby, discover that these feelings are not as frightening as he, in his own aloneness, had feared them to be." The program began in 1968 with a grant from the Hogg Foundation and did not rely on regularly budgeted university funds; thus, as a volunteer handbook stated, it was "separate from the 'establishment,' yet it allow[ed] it to utilize the full collaborative efforts of the Austin community." Students who called the telephone hotline at the student counseling center might be referred to The Listening Ear, whose "mobile care-giving squad" could travel to a caller's residence or any local place where they might be needed to "talk to a distressed person," "listen sympathetically," or make a referral to other services.

Staffed with student volunteers under the direction of a psychologist, The Listening Ear symbolized the goals of the community mental health movement. It brought mental health out of the hospital, and even out of the clinic, into more everyday settings. Small in scale, such interventions evoked the brand of "positive mental health" that had been the byword of the mental hygiene movement at the start of the twentieth century and that the Hogg Foundation had promoted through its circuit riding lectures around Texas in the 1940s and 1950s. The Listening Ear also built on the campaign to reform and then limit the use of large, stigmatized institutions in the treatment of people with mental illness. During the 1960s, the impersonal university had occupied a similar institutionalized space in the imaginations of mental health reformers, leading to the development of student counseling services as well as innovative services offered in informal settings such as coffee shops or even more personalized locations such as an individual's residence.

Reflecting on the pace of change in 1967, Foundation director Sutherland wondered:

> Must we always go through the crude cycle of a "traumatic experience," like the Whitman case, to bring an awakening to obvious problems; then experience a sudden surge of interest and a remarkable unanimity of purpose; and then become slightly disillusioned when progress slows, interest wanes, and jurisdictional squabbles arise? Is such inching ahead through a series of peaks and valleys the nature of change? Or, is there really such a thing as a "breakthrough" or as "steady progress"?[88]

The Foundation would confront such questions as it entered a new era, with new leadership, after having seemingly achieved most of its major goals in mental health reform.

6

The Unfinished Revolution, 1970–2000

Over his mild objections, Robert L. Sutherland was honored at an afternoon barbeque held on October 18, 1970, at Ima Hogg's family plantation home in Winedale, cohosted by Harry Ransom, chancellor of the University of Texas System. The occasion was Sutherland's recent retirement as the inaugural head of the Hogg Foundation for Mental Health, a position he had held for almost exactly thirty years.[1] From around Texas and the nation, luminaries in the fields of mental health and philanthropy paid tribute to Sutherland. "The wisdom of our choice has been demonstrated again and again," recalled former University of Texas president Homer Rainey, writing in a memorial book produced for the occasion.[2] According to Ima, "all concerned [had] reason to be proud" of Sutherland's tenure.[3] Many of Sutherland's oldest colleagues wrote heartfelt messages to him. Ernest E. Neal, the former Prairie View A&M University professor who had served as consultant for the Foundation's project in Slocum in the late 1940s, "relived my long years of association with you and with the Hogg Foundation" upon receiving a copy of the memorial book in the mail. "The book is a testimony to a completely dedicated man who had the insight and ability to make the Hogg Foundation a reality," Neal gushed. "This letter is my testimonial to one of the rarest, most insightful, and successful men it has been my privilege to know."[4] Longtime collaborator Loyd Rowland of the Louisiana Association for Mental Health wrote to Bernice Moore, "I think the morale of the Hogg Foundation is the highest of any group I have ever known, and I think that is something you and Bob have brought about because of your sincere devotion to things that matter."[5]

By the time of Sutherland's retirement, the "things that mattered" in mental health looked drastically different than they had in 1940. At both the federal and state levels, entire agencies devoted comparatively vast budgetary resources to the provision of mental health services, the support of basic and applied research related to mental health and mental illness, the training of mental health service providers, and the promulgation of public education on mental health. The state's leading public universities had developed undergraduate and graduate programs in psychiatry, psychology, social work, and other fields closely related to mental health. They also had begun to take seriously the provision of counseling services to their student, staff, and faculty populations. Similarly, at the local level, public and private agencies began to offer a range of mental health services, inspired by the community mental health movement and supported by newly available funding sources. No longer the sole actor on the scene, the Hogg Foundation was free to devote its resources to supporting innovative start-up and demonstration programs outside of the sudden plethora of established agencies and institutions. Many of these programs offered innovations in service delivery methods for historically underserved populations in impoverished rural or urban areas.

The Foundation's revised emphasis responded to the demands of more militant civil rights organizations for higher levels of social services in minority communities, at a time when President Lyndon Johnson's War on Poverty was directing unprecedented levels of federal funds for those services. Historians have documented how city governments and civil rights groups clashed over the appropriate usage of those funds, as well as control over the programs they were intended to support.[6] These struggles often developed along a triangular pattern of conflict that included local elected officials, usually white and politically conservative, who equated community empowerment with lawlessness; white liberal academics and experts, many of whom brought technocratic assumptions of cultural superiority to their tasks; and nonwhite community residents, who sought self-determination and were suspicious of the motives of outsiders to their communities. In Texas, antipoverty programs became one of several focal points for the Chicano movement that emerged in the late 1960s and early 1970s.[7] Founded in San Antonio in 1967, the Mexican American Youth Organization led campaigns against discrimination in voting, schooling, housing, and the distribution of resources and services throughout South Texas and other parts of the southwest United States. The organization eventually gave way, in 1969, to a third political party, the La Raza Unida Party (RUP), which mounted electoral campaigns for municipal and statewide office. The leaders of these organizations articulated a "Chicano" identity that drew on shared historical experiences and cultures of the United States–Mexico borderlands region and demanded political, social, and cultural equality with the Anglo population of the region. Although it was an identity-based social movement that broke dramatically with the more assimilationist Mexican American civil rights movement that had preceded it, the Chicano movement called for similar legal, political, and economic demands but did so in a more militant, assertive tone. The movement swept across South Texas during the 1960s, as labor strikes, boycotts, protest marches, and student walkouts at high schools and colleges challenged a range of discriminatory practices. In Texas cities, local Chicano civil rights groups insisted on equal access to social services made available by the War on Poverty, as well as a say in how those services would be constructed and distributed. As we shall see, these currents presented the Foundation with a drastically changed social and political landscape for its community mental health grants program and particularly for its interest in working with minority groups whose views of their own needs might differ from those of staff members at the Foundation.[8]

Sutherland's successor and former associate director, Wayne Holtzman, who officially assumed the role of president of the Hogg Foundation in September 1970, was the individual who crafted and carried forward the Foundation's new agenda. During the preceding decade, Holtzman's career path had taken him away from the Foundation. After a one-year fellowship at Stanford University, Holtzman had returned to the University of Texas to become dean of the College of Education in 1964. For the remainder of that decade, Holtzman served as a sometime consultant to the Foundation and editor of the Foundation's research monograph series while holding an endowed faculty position as Hogg Professor of Psychology and Education. In early 1970, Sutherland approached Holtzman about taking over the leadership of the Foundation. The pair had numerous conversations, many of them outdoor "hilltop conferences" near Sutherland's home in west Austin. By this time, Holtzman had established a vast network of federal, state, and private grant-making agencies, which he had been mining to develop new programs at the College of Education. He had built a national and international reputation in the field of psychology with his inkblot perception and personality protocol and had held administrative positions with nearly every major national and regional professional organization in psychology. Moreover, Holtzman had built cross-border partnerships with mental health researchers in Mexico and Latin America, forecasting a growing hemispheric focus for the Foundation. Thus, in Sutherland's view, Holtzman was a good choice as successor, as a longtime collaborator in the Foundation's work and a well-connected and respected mental health expert in his own right.[9]

Holtzman inherited a Foundation whose focus had shifted in the preceding half-decade toward providing grants-in-aid to local and regional start-up and pilot programs. In 1965 the Foundation began to devote about half of its annual budget to the "encouragement and testing of new patterns in mental health education and community action"; the following year, it further defined its "role of 'convener' or stimulator of groups of people from various organizations," as "specialized distributor" of ideas to local groups, "referral agent" for groups seeking resources, "initiator and 'planter' of seed ideas," and "collaborator in mental health planning."[10] In Holtzman's first year as president, the Foundation funded a range of pilot or start-up programs, both at the University of Texas and in local communities, typically for a duration of about three years with the idea that Foundation seed grants would lead to a more stable funding arrangement. For instance, the Foundation supported a vocational rehabilitation program for individuals with schizophrenia in Big Spring, a parent education project in Houston, a visiting social worker program in El Paso, a clinical consultant program in the Dallas Independent School District, and a planning grant for a community mental health center in Bexar County (San Antonio).[11] Such grants were often awarded to university departments, local or state public agencies, or private nonprofit organizations. Over the course of Holtzman's tenure as president (and later executive director) of the Foundation until 1993, this grants program would become the Foundation's primary activity. However, as Holtzman assumed the presidency, the most pressing issue facing the Foundation concerned access to mental health services for historically disadvantaged populations such as African Americans and Mexican Americans.

Mental Health and "Those Population Groups"

Always a part of its program, the Foundation's work in African American and Mexican American communities began to expand in the 1960s. In particular, the Foundation began to focus on the historically underserved South Texas region, which was the only part of the state to record no mental health clinics or psychological services in the surveys completed earlier that decade as part of the Texas Plan for Mental Health (see chapter 5). Holtzman's own interest in the region had grown out of his research collaborations with social and behavioral scientists from the region as well as from Mexico. Between 1957 and 1961, the Foundation supported the Hidalgo Project on Differential Culture Change and Mental Health, a study of "folk customs, social organization, medical practices and beliefs in the lower Rio Grande Valley" conducted by a team of American and Mexican anthropologists.[12] The study's conclusions, summarized in a preface written by Holtzman, recommended cooperation between "modern" psychologists and psychiatrists and traditional *curanderos* (folk medicine healers) relied upon by many Mexican American residents of the Valley. Of the study's fourteen recommendations, nearly all of them emphasized respect for traditional folkways and the use of bilingual professional staff, preferably of Mexican or Mexican American ancestry.[13] Around this same time, Holtzman was engaged in other cross-border studies that would be published a few years later as part of the Foundation's research monograph series. Two of the final publications in the series, *Delinquency in Three Cultures* (1969) and *Personality in Two Cultures* (1975), expanded on some of the questions raised in the Hidalgo County study. Holtzman supervised the publication of the first study and coauthored the second one along with Rogelio Díaz-Guerrero, a psychology professor at the National University of Mexico.

Delinquency in Three Cultures drew on data gathered between 1959 and 1961 from a pool of three hundred teenage boys ages thirteen to seventeen years old. The boys were broken into three groups, demarcated by ethnicity and national origin; hence the "three cultures": Mexican boys in Monterrey, Mexican American boys in San Antonio, and Anglo boys in San Antonio. All of the boys came from working-class neighborhoods; researchers located half of the boys in each cohort through the local juvenile court and the other half through the neighborhood high school.[14] A research team, led by sociologist Carl Rosenquist, administered a series of standardized intelligence and psychological tests. These tests suffered from language barriers; some of them were available only in English and were administered orally by bilingual research assistants.[15] In addition, lead researcher Rosenquist misplaced a large number of the individual interview notes during a move from Texas to California. The task of finishing the manuscript thus fell to Edwin Megargee, a colleague of Wayne Holtzman in the psychology department at the University of Texas. Although the data suggested complex differences between delinquent and nondelinquent boys and between the three "cultural" groups, Megargee concluded that similar factors caused delinquency across the three groups. He identified a similar inability to defer gratification, lowered expectations for the future, and a lack of home stability, all features that figured prominently in the then-influential theory of a "culture of poverty" articulated by anthropologist Oscar Lewis in his studies of poor families in Latin America, Mexico, and the United States.[16] Indeed, an advertisement touted the book as a pioneering cross-cultural study that promised to explain the causes of delinquency among teenagers from the "culture of poverty." A longitudinal research model formed the basis for *Personality in Two Cultures* (1975), which surveyed six sets of 800 schoolchildren in Austin and Mexico City in staggered three-year intervals over a six-year period.[17] Relying on the Holtzman Inkblot Technique and other testing protocols, the study presented thorough empirical findings in contrast to the partial data in *Delinquency in Three Cultures.* Although their critical reception was mixed, these two studies were noteworthy as transitional documents in the history of mental health. They suggested how the field was becoming more interested in Mexican American, Mexican-origin, and Latin American populations. At the same time, as we shall see, these anthropologically influenced studies tended to produce uneasy relationships between largely Anglo mental health experts and officials and the nonwhite communities in which they conducted studies or established mental health services.[18]

The focus on nonwhite populations extended beyond these research projects. In 1969 the Foundation was supporting more than thirty community projects addressing mental health needs of African American and Mexican American populations. The broad spectrum of regions and services ranged from rural public health clinics in East Texas to school counseling programs in San Antonio and El Paso high schools.[19] In 1970, Holtzman's first year as president, the Foundation announced that it was devoting "extra attention" to "the problems of special minority groups," convening a "Congress of Black Professionals in Higher Education" and initiating a three-year demonstration project that would open a community mental health clinic to serve the Mexican American population of Crystal City in south Texas.[20] The new approach reflected the input from the Foundation's National Advisory Council, which during the 1960s included such luminaries as Robert Felix, former National Institute of Mental Health director; Bertram Brown, National Institute of Mental Health director; philanthropist Jeanette Rockefeller, president of the National Association for Mental Health; psychiatrist Howard Rome, president of the American Psychiatric Association; psychologist Nicholas Hobbs, president of the American Psychological Association; and Homer Wadsworth, head of the Kansas City School Board and later the Cleveland Foundation.[21] At its December 1968 meeting, the advisory council's message to the Foundation was that it should focus on voids overlooked by the new community mental health centers. In the council's view, the Texas Department of Mental Health and Mental Retardation (TDMHMR) appeared to be shifting former hospital patients ("hard core, chronic patients") to the new mental health centers, inhibiting its ability to fulfill its potential for offering more broadly available treatment services. The Foundation not only needed to support programs that filled these unmet needs but to pilot cooperative projects that brought together white and nonwhite professionals with nonwhite community groups.[22] At the following year's council meeting, Ira Iscoe wondered aloud whether "the Hogg Foundation should be on the lookout for unusual or 'far out' projects" that would "challenge the 'power structure'" while also bringing mental health services to underserved populations.[23] This vague notion seemed to crystallize during an afternoon presentation on the needs of Mexican Americans given by a team that included Guadalupe Zamarripa, president of the university chapter of the Mexican American Youth Organization. "There are no adapted methods for teaching Mexican Americans," admonished Zamarripa, who seems to have made a major impression on the advisory council. "Traditional methods of teaching first-graders are Anglo and are not in the context of the needs of Mexican American children. We need more progressiveness in bilingual education, up to and through the secondary school level."[24] These discussions came to a head at the January

1971 council meeting, which focused entirely on "ethnic group dilemmas."[25] Identity-based social movements had given rise to a plethora of nonprofits run by and for nonwhite populations, in many cases attempting to provide services that were broadly defined and sometimes led by individuals who were not social service professionals. These "nontraditional agencies" were submitting grant requests to the Foundation that were "related to minority group problems with only the minimum of descriptive information and little or no budget analysis."[26]

Moreover, the Foundation confronted "the growing attitude among some more militant leaders among both Chicanos and Blacks that they be given grants, unstructured and with little or no outline of operating procedures, on the premise that 'only Chicanos can know Chicano needs,' or 'only Blacks can know and, therefore, meet Black requirements.'"[27] Were the Foundation to respond as it typically would have in past years to such unstructured proposals, yet another problem arose:

> There is a need for our understanding a proposal from a minority group when it is placed in such simple language as would be definitive. We need the imagination to know that some applicants cannot articulate in such a way as to appeal to us: that back of this, with some imagination, can be found a proposal. Also our replies may be so cluttered with terminology that we understand (like innovative, replicative, evaluation, etc.) that recipients tend not to understand our basis for reply; rather to feel that they are turned down because they are a minority group.[28]

These sorts of conflicts echoed those playing out in antipoverty projects in inner-city neighborhoods across the nation. Such misunderstandings could be exacerbated when it came to community mental health initiatives in this period. In spite of the Foundation's historically expansive definition of mental health, which had incorporated infrastructure needs similar to those identified by antipoverty projects, it struggled to work effectively with minority communities. One solution emerged from the January 1971 advisory council meeting: hire professional staff from the same racial and ethnic backgrounds as the communities the Foundation hoped to serve.[29] The idea was proposed by two new members of the Foundation's advisory council: Rogelio Diaz-Guerrero, Mexican psychiatry professor and Holtzman research partner, and Claudio Arenas, architecture professor at the University of Texas. Noting that "Chicano groups" would need assistance formulating grant proposals but would not want that help directly from Foundation staff as currently constituted, they suggested the use of "a liaison person" who was "already familiar with their needs."[30] Such proposals should be evaluated for more than their immediate impact:

> Their needs should be expressed by themselves, no matter how unsophisticated that expression, and if necessary interpreted by someone who understands what they are saying. . . . grant to an ethnic group . . . is a transfer of a resource which, in reality, is a transfer of power and indication of concern. The amount of funds the Foundation has is small compared to the need. He suggested that perhaps the Foundation in making grants should think more of transferring the symbolism that there is real care and concern rather than concentrating on finding a break-through project. The risks may be high, but the possibilities for attitudinal changes are great.[31]

It was around this time that the Foundation hired its first Mexican American and African American professional staff members: Adrian Fowler, assigned to work with black communities largely in the Austin, Houston, and Dallas-Fort Worth metropolitan areas, and Reymundo Rodríguez, assigned to the sprawling, predominantly Mexican and Mexican American region of South Texas. The pair brought eclectic personal and professional backgrounds to the Foundation. Fowler, who held degrees in biology and animal science, was a graduate of historically black Huston-Tillotson College in east Austin.[32] Rodríguez, on the other hand, had taken a somewhat circuitous route to the Foundation. A native of Eagle Pass in South Texas, Rodriguez held degrees in health science and urban planning from Texas A&M University. Prior to joining the Foundation, he had worked as an intern at a psychiatric unit in a Houston veteran's hospital, as a schoolteacher in the same elementary school he had attended in Eagle Pass, and as an official in the Council of Governments for a nine-county region in South Texas.[33] "Before Adrian and Reymundo were hired, the staff was all Anglo," recalled longtime Foundation staff member Ralph Culler. By the 1970s, "there was a strong interest in the Foundation to focus on minorities."[34] Rodríguez, who joined the Foundation in 1971, "came on because [Foundation president] Holtzman said, 'I want to focus on South Texas. I want to focus on Mexican-Americans, Chicanos . . . I want to focus on those population groups. And I want you to go out there and do training, technical assistance, and bring me some proposals that are good, that are fundable, that are well-written, that have a good evaluation component.'"[35] Rodríguez's baptism of fire would come in his first major project, located in one of the nerve centers of the Mexican American civil rights movement: Crystal City in Zavala County.

The Case of Cristal: Bringing Mental Health Services to the Rio Grande Valley

On February 19, 1971, about three weeks after the aforementioned advisory council meeting, Robert Sutherland and a team of faculty from the University of Texas Health Science Center (UTHSC) in San Antonio drove down to Crystal City to meet with leaders of the RUP.[36] The meeting had been arranged by Sally Jones Andrade, a research assistant in the psychology department at UTHSC, whose husband Erasmo Andrade was a longtime activist in the Mexican American civil rights movement. In the 1960s, he had chaired the Valley Workers Assistance Committee, which helped support farm workers' strikes in the Rio Grande Valley, and in the year prior to the Foundation meeting, had worked closely with teacher's groups on integration of the region's public schools.[37] That same year, the RUP had ousted a long entrenched Anglo minority from political power by winning the local school board and city elections in three cities of the Winter Garden area in South Texas. Notably, one of the RUP's founders and its leader, José Angel Gutiérrez, had been elected president of the Crystal City school board in 1970. Like Gutiérrez, the RUP leadership was comprised mainly of young, educated Mexican Americans from South Texas who had developed sophisticated critiques not only of the Anglo-dominated "power structure" but also of liberal organizations such as the Hogg Foundation, which activists viewed as part of that same structure.[38] In his 1974 book, *A Gringo Manual on How to Handle Mexicans*, Gutiérrez described their preliminary meetings with the Hogg Foundation specifically to illustrate how foundations "say one thing and do another" and "shrug off their responsibility" to treat Mexican American grant applicants fairly.[39] He called this technique "throwing out the bone," predicated on a "well known *gringo* stereotype" that Chicanos will squabble among themselves and thus sabotage their prospects for obtaining funds:

> In 1970, the Hogg Foundation of Texas announced the availability of funds for a Chicano mental health project. Groups of Chicanos from throughout the state met for the purpose of soliciting money. The Foundation people threw out the bone. "Whichever group the people assembled here can agree on, will get the funds," they said. They expected a big fight. The groups promptly voted that all monies go to Cristal. There was no fight. A caucus had been held previous to the meeting where agreement was reached.[40]

RUP suspicions notwithstanding, the meeting made a profound impression on Sutherland, who found the scenes of "dismal poverty" in Crystal City appalling. "Crystal City is another world," he reflected later. "Seeing it is not enough to believe it."[41] Both Sutherland and the UTHSC team felt that "nothing short of a coordinated and broad program" that included public health "would make a significant difference."[42] They also agreed that the social and political changes taking place were promising and scheduled a second meeting for March 4, 1971, in a community center in a west side *barrio* neighborhood of San Antonio. At this meeting with "about a dozen Chicano leaders from South Texas," Foundation president Holtzman faced a more openly skeptical reception. Some of the Chicano leaders told Holtzman that they knew the Foundation only as "the funder of Anglo anthropological studies which perpetuated a stereotypic, assimilationist view of the Mexican American." Andrade recalled that another attendee from Crystal City confided to her that they hoped to "pick up some bread" from "a white institution that they felt had never met its responsibility to Chicanos." In Holtzman's recollection, Gutiérrez told the group that "[n]one of you guys are going to ever do anything for Chicanos." Holtzman took this skepticism to heart. "And that's when I said—I swore to him . . . [that] we were going to set up this clinic in Crystal City, and we were going to provide mental health services to a lot of people in South Texas." The response, "I'll believe it when I see it," set forth a challenge the Foundation accepted.[43] It agreed to a modest five-year grant of $35,000, as well as the formation of a Chicano Advisory Board and the employment of a "Chicano professional" to serve as a liaison to the Crystal City project.[44] The Foundation responded to the third condition by recruiting Reymundo Rodríguez, who had attended the initial planning meeting in Crystal City while still an employee of the Council of Governments, without his employer's permission "on my own dime" as he recounted it:

> I met Dr. Holtzman and [Stan Brown, Foundation staff member] in Crystal City. We had a conversation about the application that was submitted to fund a community health clinic in Crystal City. I was not given permission by my employer to attend. I did attend. Dr. Holtzman called me a couple of days later and asked me if I wanted to come work at the Hogg Foundation for Mental Health. He asked me to come visit him in Austin, which I did on a weekend. We got together and we talked. I told him at the time that I had always dreamed of getting a college credential and going back to work with the people I knew and loved. His response to me was that if I came to work with him, that I could help more people throughout the State of Texas, including the people I knew and loved. He also said that being an integral part of the University of Texas, we would be based on campus and that I might be able to pursue a Ph.D. or continue my education. So I came up. I thought that Dr. Holtzman was somebody who was very personable. I had read some of the articles concerning the Rorschach ink blot technique, which had now been advanced and also tested cross culturally. His book was translated into eight languages . . . he had a lot of appreciation for the language and the culture. Not that he would have a very deep understanding of Mexico or Mexican Americans as a homogeneous group, but that he understood the heterogeneity of the Hispanic populations in Texas, in Mexico, and Latin America. That impressed me.[45]

The Zavala County Mental Health Project, so named to avoid a direct association with the politically unpopular Crystal City, struggled mightily during its five-year existence. Local white officials and businessmen uniformly opposed the provision of any funds to the RUP regime. After the 1972 gubernatorial election, won by Democrat Dolph Briscoe of nearby Uvalde, the RUP faced a hostile state administration as well; Briscoe nearly had lost the election due to the RUP's third-party challenge, and he famously had referred to Crystal City as "little Cuba." Moreover, TDMHMR expressed displeasure with the Foundation for funding the mental health project without involving the agency, despite the state's historical lack of involvement in providing mental health services to the region. Indeed, "stimulating the interest of TDMHMR" was one of the Foundation's unofficial goals for the project.[46]

Shifting political alliances within the Chicano movement and the RUP also undermined the project, with "maybe five political factions" competing with one another in Crystal City alone throughout the period; according to Foundation staffer Rodríguez, "everything was politicized."[47] Political infighting affected the mental health project because the Foundation acceded to the demand for local control; the project director and much of the top staff reported to city and county officials. As a result, the five-year grant period witnessed four different directors presiding over the mental health project. The first of those directors was Erasmus Andrade, who established public health services through the Hogg Foundation grant as well as additional federal and state funds awarded by the Office of Economic Opportunity, the National Institute of Mental Health, and the Texas Department of Welfare. Mental health services were provided by visiting teams from UTHSC (led by Mexican American psychiatrist Cervanto Martinez Jr.), along with local paraprofessionals who received training from UTHSC psychology and psychiatry faculty. These latter-day mental health "circuit riders" commuted weekly between San Antonio and the three-county Winter Garden region in the Valley during the 1970s. However, Andrade left the directorship after two years to run for public office; his successor lacked professional qualifications and appears to have been appointed due to his political connections—a recurring problem for the project, from the Foundation's perspective. Under the new direction, the project drifted away from its mental health focus and became "a general social services agency with a definitive welfare orientation."[48] Nevertheless, the project achieved some successes: greater investment from TDMHMR, mainly in the form of visiting outpatient services from staff at the San Antonio State Hospital; in-service trainings tailored for Chicano paraprofessionals from a "*barrio* consultant" in west San Antonio; and, in May 1976, the opening of the Centro de Salud (community health center) in Crystal City. Providing a range of health services that included mental health, the center opened two years behind schedule due largely to political infighting that saw the second director and much of his staff removed amid charges of financial improprieties.

Andrade's final assessment of the project, written in 1978, was mixed. On the one hand, as psychiatrist Martinez put it, "clinical psychiatric services had been regularly provided for seven years to low-income, Spanish-speaking, emotionally disturbed individuals in a town 120 miles away from the nearest State facility."[49] The involvement of the San Antonio State Hospital helped spur TDMHMR to increase appropriations for community mental health services in South Texas, nearly doubling its number of funded staff positions from thirty-six to seventy-three. However, the project's most tangible goal, the development of a community mental health center, was never fully realized; the Centro de Salud offered a limited range of mental health services as part of a comprehensive community health clinic. Similarly, the project's broader aims at cultural change around mental health seemed only partially achieved. The project had aspired to destigmatize mental illness and to habituate the local population to the use of mental health services. Although the project reported sizable if intermittent caseloads, several residents reportedly viewed the health center mainly as a source of pharmaceutical medications ("a pill shop," as some told Andrade). As initial funding and activity levels tapered off in the late 1970s, many residents reverted back to what had been the traditional practice of traveling to Mexico to obtain health services. Initially focused on children, youth, and individuals with substance abuse issues, the project by its conclusion found itself treating a client base that was largely older, many of them recent discharges from the state hospital. Although "lofty promises" were not quite met, the project nevertheless did provide "a diversity of services" and "a place to go without fear," according to one resident.[50]

Andrade's final assessment included a discussion of the crucial role of "cultural brokers"—essentially, mental health professionals who were either bilingual or of Mexican or Mexican American origin. These brokers often found themselves caught between the expectations of ethnic and political loyalties to the Chicano movement, and the accompanying suspicions of *gringo* individuals and organizations, and the professional standards of foundations, government agencies, and mental health fields. Jobs formed the most obvious arena of conflict between these two broad imperatives; RUP officials reportedly expected that political loyalists would be hired for positions regardless of their qualifications, putting "cultural brokers" in the uncomfortable position of upholding professional standards at the cost of their personal relationships in the community. Even an experienced broker, such as Foundation staffer Rodríguez, struggled to overcome this conflict. Rodríguez had functioned in this capacity as a staff member in the regional

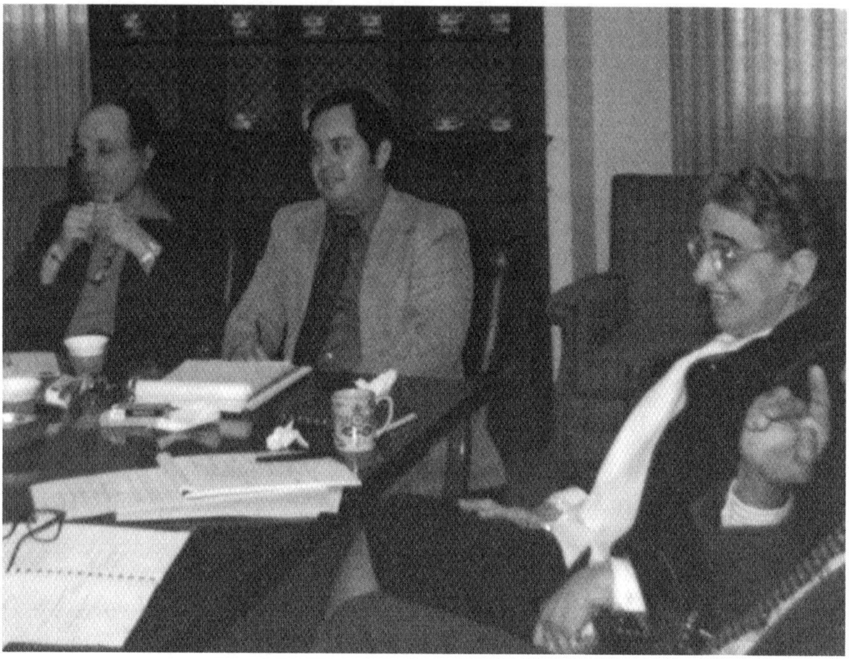

6.1. Reymundo Rodriguez (center) at a National Advisory Council meeting, spring 1976. Box MAI9-U136, Hogg Foundation Papers.

Council of Governments prior to joining the Zavala County Mental Health Outreach Project, working with Anglo law enforcement officials and Mexican American residents. Accusations of "selling out" were "very common, even when I came to the Hogg Foundation," recalled Rodriguez. "And yet, the thing was, 'Hey, give me a grant.' Me: 'Write a proposal.' Them: 'Why? You're there. Get me a grant.' Me: 'Well, I can't just get you a grant.' Them: 'Well, why not? Did you sell out?'"[51] At the same time, the project demonstrated the need to do more than simply expand existing service models to underserved communities; those models had to change to meet distinctive community needs. In the case of Cristal, that primarily meant Spanish-speaking and Mexican American service providers and the provision of more "culturally appropriate" services that took family and community into account more fully.[52]

Even as the Crystal City project unfolded, the Hogg Foundation began reporting its allocation of grant dollars to minority applicants during its national advisory council meetings. For instance, during the 1973–74 fiscal year, the Crystal City grant was by far the Foundation's largest award. Mexican American communities comprised about one-fifth of all grant-funded projects, with African Americans at 7 percent and "general" comprising the remainder.[53] This trend in the Foundation's expenditures reflected a growing national concern about access to mental health services for historically underserved populations. However, it also placed the Foundation in a unique position during the 1980s and 1990s, a time when the state and national landscape for mental health underwent new changes.

"A Totally Different Game Now": The Convener Foundation in the 1980s and 1990s

On February 17, 1977, President Jimmy Carter issued an executive order creating the President's Commission on Mental Health. The commission was tasked with proposing solutions to a mental health system that had fallen into disarray over the preceding decade due to a host of national and state policy shifts. Along with the development of community mental health centers in the 1960s, federal entitlements such as Medicare, Medicaid, Social Security Disability Insurance, Supplemental Security Income, food stamps, and housing supports had enabled a range of individuals with mental illness to reside in community rather than institutional settings. In addition, the growth of employer-sponsored health insurance after World War II provided individuals with some access to mental health services. In response to these developments, state governments (including Texas, as we have seen) began moving individuals out of large institutions such as state hospitals and special schools and into community settings such as group homes, assisted-living facilities, and private residences supported by a range of services.[54] As a result, by the late 1970s, the mental health system included "a bewildering variety of institutions" whose disorganization allowed numerous individuals with mental illness to slip through the cracks, sometimes turning up in homeless shelters.[55] Moreover, this confused state of affairs disproportionately affected communities of color. Thus the President's Commission was tasked with devising "a unified approach to all mental health and people-helping services," identifying underserved groups and ways to provide services to them, and parsing out the appropriate roles for the federal, state, local, and private sectors.[56]

Out of a list of more than one thousand nominees, twenty commissioners were selected whose interests "revolved around the mental health needs of minorities and underserved groups." Among the chosen commissioners was the Hogg Foundation's own Reymundo Rodríguez. The commission received reports from over two dozen separate "task panels" involving 250 individuals, providing research-based recommendations on numerous topics related to mental health. In addition, the commission held four public hearings in different locations around the country. During the summer and fall of 1977, the commission met to assimilate the findings of the task panels and the hearings and found itself confronted with a confusing array of issues. A tension emerged between psychiatric and nonpsychiatric issues; most of the commissioners were not psychiatrists or psychologists and had not worked directly in the delivery or administration of mental health treatment, while many of the individuals who provided research through the task panels and the public hearings were academic or professional experts. Thus the commission's final report, presented to President Carter in April 1978, emphasized "societal ills," as well as psychiatric causes for mental illness, and included a long and comprehensive list of recommendations. The two major areas of agreement on the commission focused on the need to provide access to mental health services for underserved populations and to improve services for individuals with serious mental illness who required additional supports such as housing and general health services.[57]

In response to the President's Commission report, the Texas Senate created a Special Committee on the Delivery of Human Services to evaluate steps toward meeting the report's recommendations. The Foundation awarded a two-year grant of $71,500 to Citizens for Human Development, a "grassroots citizen effort" whose purpose was to provide recommendations to the special committee. Citizens for Human Development sent a newsletter to seven thousand people, conducted an opinion survey of about two thousand service professionals, and conducted public forums to discuss its findings, which were described as "input to the various planning bodies currently affecting mental health and mental retardation expenditures from the local level to the state level." In 1982 this initiative gave way to a Mental Health Code Task Force, funded by a Foundation grant while it developed recommendations for revising the code.[58] In 1985 the legislature adopted wide-ranging revisions, including a requirement that all community mental health centers (CMHCs) provide services regardless of ability to pay; new requirements for the TDMHMR to provide services in all regions of the state; and permission for the TDMHMR to contract with private providers if necessary to fulfill its mandate. A host of other changes addressed voluntary and involuntary commitment proceedings and removed outdated terminology from existing statutes.[59]

At the federal level, the President's Commission report spurred the passage of new major legislation, the Mental Health Systems Act of 1980, which attempted to address both of those aforementioned areas. It provided grants to CMHCs to encourage expanded services to underserved and higher-need populations, as well as funds for a host of other mental health initiatives. However, the law was repealed barely a year after its passage by the newly elected administration of President Ronald Reagan in 1981. In addition, Reagan's first budget converted an array of federally funded mental health programs, including CMHCs, into block grants awarded to states to use as they wished with few restrictions and sharply reduced overall federal funding for mental health. As a result, in the 1980s, state mental health agencies suddenly found themselves stripped of funds and therefore unable to fulfill the mandates from President Carter's commission, particularly in the provision of services to historically underserved populations. A further change took place in the early 1990s with the advent of managed care in the private insurance system and subsequently in Medicaid, which decentralized and privatized the management of mental health services in the name of containing costs.[60]

The sudden downturn in public funding for mental health services during the Reagan years placed the Hogg Foundation in a "reactive rather than proactive" position, fielding a slew of grant requests from community mental health agencies and nonprofits.[61] The result was a narrowing of Foundation activities; ambitious research and public policy initiatives that were once central gave way to an expanded array of small-scale grants. The Foundation made some grant funds available to local and state governmental agencies such as the TDMHMR but seems to have worked in a limited consulting capacity with these agencies. For instance, in 1982–83 the Foundation awarded grants to the TDMHMR ($14,000) and the Texas Mental Health Association ($17,918) for the purpose of revising the state's mental health code, which the Foundation had supported and even agitated for in its initial iteration in 1957. A more representative award came the following year, when the Foundation supported a TDMHMR pilot program that provided "adjunctive support for case managers and their clients at six community MHMR [Mental Health Mental Retardation] centers."[62] These sorts of grants seemed more clearly to be filling voids left by a lack of adequate public funding.

Around this time, an internal debate appears to have ensued about the extent to which the Foundation's mission was fulfilling the wishes of Ima Hogg and the Hogg family. Annual reports in the 1980s began to invoke "donor intent," seemingly to explain a shift in budgetary expenditures away from research and public policy and toward categories labeled "service delivery" and "program development."[63] By this time, neither Ima Hogg nor Robert Sutherland was alive to comment, having passed away in 1975 and 1976, respectively; moreover, the final installment in the Hogg Foundation research monograph series had quietly been discontinued. Some staff worried about "antipathy between scholarship and science on the one side and service and advocacy on the other." The Foundation's 1982 annual report proposed this resolution: "All research, all science, all scholarship are an investment in future service, and all present day service is a reflection of that past investment in science and scholarship. There should be some balance, some proportion between them."[64] As a result, throughout the 1980s and 1990s, the Foundation gradually devoted the bulk of its resources to its evaluation research program, which Holtzman had launched in 1974.[65] In this model, evaluation research associates solicited, supervised, and evaluated grant proposals developed by fledgling and more established nonprofit groups in local communities. Ideally, the Foundation awarded startup grants to programs that promised innovation in mental health service construction or delivery or introduced services to previously underserved populations. One of those evaluation research consultants, Ralph Culler, was a graduate of Ira Iscoe's program in community psychology at the University of Texas, where he enrolled in courses on program evaluation. In 1975 Culler became one of the first graduate students to be awarded an evaluation research fellow at the Foundation. The fellowship led to a permanent position as an evaluation research associate assigned to the Houston–Harris County region, where Culler supervised grants awarded under the Ima Hogg Foundation, a separate endowment created in 1964 and activated shortly after her death in 1975 to support children's mental health in Ima's home region. For instance, starting in 1984, the Ima Hogg Foundation supported the Casa de Esperanza de Los Ninos, a postadoption program for young children with disabilities, including HIV. Founded in 1982 on a shoestring budget, the Casa de Esperanza relied on Foundation funds through much of the 1980s and early 1990s. Today, it has a $3 million annual operating budget. Culler called his work with Casa de Esperanza "some of the most rewarding work" of his career.[66]

In 1987 the Foundation began a three-year initiative intended to commemorate the fiftieth anniversary of its founding by assembling three commissions to mount major studies of mental health. The approach broadly resembled that of the President's Commission on Mental Health, although in this case sprung from a private foundation rather than a government entity. The Commissions on Community Care of the Mentally Ill, the Mental Health of Children and Their Families, and the Mental Health of Adolescents and Young Adults gathered information over three years (1987–90) and were comprised of public- and private-sector professionals, including Foundation staff. Findings were presented at symposia and in numerous publications, including resource books and policy proposals, and received some attention from the local news media. The immediate effect of the Commission reports was that they laid some groundwork for the inauguration of the Foundation's School of the Future program, a statewide demonstration project that ran from 1992 to 1997. With a budget of about $2 million, the Foundation identified inner-city public schools in Austin, Dallas, Houston, and San Antonio that would serve as laboratories for the integration of children's mental health services into the school's program. Its premise was that, in poor communities, the public school should serve as a center for health and human services as well as for education—an idea then endorsed by the American Psychological Association and being tested in other parts of the country. The project introduced a range of services, including school psychologists, family counseling services, and substance abuse programs, many of which would go on to become regularly funded parts of the operating budgets of public schools. In addition, the School of the Future sought to elicit greater parent involvement through a range of extracurricular programs. However, this ambitious project yielded unclear long-term results; as Ralph Culler recalled about the project sites in Houston, an extensive survey of attitudes, grades, and disciplinary reports demonstrated little measurable changes resulting from the new services. "[A]t the end of the day, however, the project did bring services into the schools—services that we knew would work with the kids they served, and relationships between the schools and service agencies were established."[67] Equipped with a seemingly substantial capital outlay, it nevertheless relied heavily on voluntary support from individuals, businesses, and public agencies in the demonstration areas. This seems to have resulted in mixed outcomes between specific programs as well as geographic areas, but even these conclusions are difficult to ascertain because published reports offered brief, anecdotal, and broad descriptions rather than tangible, quantitative data or evidence of lasting policy changes in the local school districts. The final report, produced in 1997, suggested that several of the pilot programs were discontinued for lack of consistent funds, while others were taken over by agencies such as Head Start, the TDMHMR, or the school district itself.[68]

The School of the Future project's duration overlapped with a change in the Foundation's executive director, as Holtzman's protégé, sociology professor, and longtime Foundation associate Charles Bonjean took over the role. Under Bonjean's direction, the Foundation continued along the course mapped out by Holtzman, focusing on its evaluation research program. Bonjean's term ended abruptly in 2002 when he became seriously ill. The Foundation's direction under Holtzman and Bonjean continued the "circuit riding" approach of earlier eras; the Foundation distributed information to the public about mental health, and it dispatched consultants around the state of Texas to assist with innovative mental health programs. However, the impact of these activities was limited by the predominance of the major mental health institutions and agencies that it had done so much to foster in previous eras. No longer was the Hogg Foundation the sole or even the leading source of information about a cutting-edge concept—mental health—about which most citizens knew little. The Foundation's most direct involvement with mental health tended to come in its evaluation research program, where it worked in advisory and evaluation capacities with nonprofit agencies, some of which grew into significant providers of mental health services. By the end of the twentieth century, large, bureaucratic state agencies such as the TDMHMR, private-sector service providers, and academic training and research programs occupied spaces that once had been inhabited largely by the Foundation. They provided public information on mental health, discussed issues relevant to mental health, and generally seized some degree of leadership in the larger field as well as various subfields. Mental health had become a crowded field, as Holtzman observed later:

> It's a totally different game now than the way it was back in the '50s and even the '60s. You've got a number of medical schools. And you've got a whole lot of PhD programs in psychology. You've got social work all over the place. If you look in the directory in Austin—there were two psychologists practicing psychology, psychological services, back in the '50s, only two. There are well over 200 now. It's more like 1,000 if you count the psychologists and related people. It takes pages and pages in the Yellow Pages of the phone book. It has changed.[69]

In a 2001 letter, director Bonjean described the Foundation's changing role in latter decades as "a convener—bringing together experts from a number of philanthropic and mental health-related organizations to share information and to collaborate on worthy projects."[70] A cursory review of that year's annual report showed a diverse range of funded projects: a study of the impact of managed care systems in the Harris County (Houston) Mental Health Mental Retardation department; research studies at the University of Texas, Baylor University, the University of Houston, and Texas A&M University; and a host of demonstration projects run by nonprofit agencies in children's mental health and social services. The Foundation supported public and private agencies alike, with emphasis areas in minority mental health and children's mental health. In some respects, these endeavors differed little from the grand campaigns of earlier years. Thanks in large part to the success of those campaigns, the Foundation found itself one of many entities in the mental health field at the end of the century. Its next chapter remained to be written.

EPILOGUE

People First

On February 24, 2004, the Hogg Foundation's newly minted executive director, King Davis, announced a new direction for the now-venerable organization. To address "serious contemporary mental health needs," the Foundation would "go beyond the traditional financial support of mental health services by establishing two new priority areas: Mental Health Services Research and Mental Health Policy and Law." The shift drew in part on Davis's recent experience serving on President George W. Bush's New Freedom Commission on Mental Health, which had reported that the American mental health system had become "fragmented, cumbersome, culturally inaccessible and lacking in evidence-based services."[1] Davis's appointment signaled a new direction in other ways; his personal and professional background differed significantly from those of his predecessors. An African American who grew up in Arkansas and Oklahoma, Davis moved to his grandparents' home in 1960 to attend California State University at Fresno, where he earned bachelor's and master's degrees in social work. During his undergraduate studies, Davis's field placements with former patients at the state hospitals ignited his interest in mental health. Upon completing his master's degree, Davis began a three-year tour as Chief of Social Work Services at Walson Army Hospital in Fort Dix, New Jersey, where he supervised a unit that provided intake and mental health services to wounded soldiers returning from Vietnam. At the urging of his commanding officer, Joe Bevilacqua, Davis decided to pursue a doctoral degree at Brandeis University. Soured on clinical work by his experiences at the hospital, Davis's interests shifted to mental health policy:

> My interest in clinical work ended in Fort Dix, because of the things that I saw. The absence of various services for soldiers who were returning, the difficulty we had in placing people in communities who had psychiatric problems; I also ran the pregnancy and adoption unit for the hospital, and

> what I saw happen to female soldiers. . . . It was a really difficult time period, and I had become probably more convinced than ever that being a clinician didn't bring great rewards for the people that we serviced, the nature of the science wasn't very good. And so, interacting with Bevilacqua and some others, convinced me that a policy school would probably be better. And Brandeis was perfect for that.[2]

In 1971 Davis completed his doctorate in social policy and management at Brandeis, which focused on African American philanthropic organizations. Over the next three decades, Davis held numerous academic and government positions, including posts as the Director of Community Mental Health (1970s) and the Commissioner of Mental Health and Mental Retardation (1990s) for the state of Virginia. In his dual roles as an agency administrator and a university professor, Davis was able to provide his students with unique insights into the worlds of community and institutional mental health services. In addition, Davis's career spanned the period of racial integration in Virginia's mental health agencies and systems; when he took his first administrative position in the early 1970s, he was the first African American to do so—a "tough" experience, in his recollection. In 1999 Davis accepted an endowed faculty position in the School of Social Work at the University of Texas, which was named for the Hogg Foundation's inaugural director, Robert Sutherland; four years later, he became the fourth executive director in the Foundation's history.[3]

Davis's arrival at the Foundation coincided with numerous shifts in the mental health field that have taken on a greater emphasis for the Foundation into the current day. Like many other human service fields, mental health has adopted "evidence-based practices," an approach that has been defined somewhat differently by the professional disciplines most associated with mental health. However, the general definition calls for mental health decision-making, policy, and practice that draw on various forms of evidence: research, clinical expertise, and individual characteristics.[4] Davis refocused the Foundation toward mental health initiatives that either drew from or contributed new knowledge to evidence-based practices: for instance, the Reducing Seclusion and Restraint program offered grant dollars to treatment centers in support of alternatives to seclusion and restraint of persons with mental illness. Noting that even evidence-based practices often proved effective only with specific segments of the population, Davis also emphasized increasing the "cultural competence" of mental health services—that is, designing and delivering services that were accessible and relevant to racial and ethnic minority populations. "In the field," observed Davis, "there really is this quest for practices that have some demonstrated outcomes based upon the method that is used."[5] During Davis's directorship, in addition to the aforementioned changes in the mental health field, one can discern a diversification not only in the demographic composition of practitioners and policymakers but in their approaches to mental health and mental illness as well. The "one-size-fits-all" approach symbolized by the asylums and mental hospitals of past eras has given way to one characterized by multiple, and often highly individualized, perspectives. Today, mental health agencies, including the Hogg Foundation, espouse "people-first" language that disavows "demeaning" labels and evinces respect for individuals with mental illness. In its use of language, and its support for mental health policies and programs that demonstrably meet "the needs of people of Texas," the Foundation has adapted its founding mission to the needs of an increasingly diverse twenty-first-century populace.[6] The humanizing impulse that drove earlier generations of circuit riders for mental health to travel the state has, for the moment, culminated in an historical moment in which academic experts and professionals seek to match their hard-won knowledge with the life experiences of the human beings they seek to help.

Notes

Introduction

1. "Father: Teen Daughter, Shot By Police, 'Should Still Be Alive,'" *San Antonio Express News*, February 9, 2015; "Answers Slow in Longview Police Department Shooting," *Marshall News Messenger*, January 23, 2015; "Texas Teen Shot Dead After Entering Station," *New York Daily News*, January 26, 2015; "Video Shows Girl Pull Knife on Texas Police Before They Shoot Her," *Los Angeles Times*, January 27, 2015; "Pared-Down City of Longview Website Online Soon," *Longview News-Journal*, February 9, 2015.

2. "17-Year-Old Girl Shot Dead by Three Cops at Texas Police Station," *Think Progress*, January 26, 2015, http://thinkprogress.org/justice/2015/01/26/3615294/kristiana-coignard-shot-cops-longview/ (accessed March 16, 2015).

3. "Longview Police Release Suicide Note of Girl Killed in Police Station," *Tyler Morning Telegraph*, April 10, 2015.

4. "Bipolar Teen's Death in Police Station Highlights Rift Between Cops, Mentally Ill," *Yahoo News*, February 5, 2015, http://news.yahoo.com/bipolar-teen-s-death-highlights-frequency-of-violent-encounters-between-police—mentally-ill-014049696.html (accessed March 16, 2015). See also "When Police Deal With People in Crisis," *CNN*, February 3, 2015, http://www.cnn.com/2015/02/03/opinion/perry-mental-illness-police/ (accessed March 17, 2015).

5. Statistics from the National Alliance on Mental Illness draw from official reports of the National Institutes of Health. "Mental Illness Facts and Numbers, 2015," National Alliance on Mental Illness www.nami.org (accessed March 18, 2015).

6. Ibid.; see also "Legislators Devote New Funding to Mental Health," *Texas Tribune*, May 19, 2013 http://www.texastribune.org/2013/05/19/transformational-funding-dedicated-mental-health/ (accessed March 20, 2015) "State Legislation Report 2013: Trends, Themes, and Best Practices in State Mental Health Legislation," October 28, 2013, www.nami.org (accessed March 20, 2015).

7. Susan Stone, *Recommendations for Updating the Texas Mental Health Code: A Response to Decades of Dramatic Change in Texas' Mental Health System* (Austin: Texas Appleseed, September 2012).

8. Edward Brown, "Moving Up Mental Health," *Fort Worth Weekly*, March 2014.

9. Stone, *Recommendations for Updating the Texas Mental Health Code*, supra note 7; see also "Protecting the Vulnerable: Texas Mental Health Code Due for an Update,"

Austin American-Statesman, January 14, 2012; "Group Discusses Statewide Mental Health Code Reform," *Odessa American*, July 25, 2011.

10. Brown, "Moving Up Mental Health," supra note 8.

11. Quoted in *A Guide to Understanding Mental Health System and Services in Texas* (Austin, TX: Hogg Foundation for Mental Health, November 2012), 125. For similar language, see the agency's mission statement, titled "Hope, Resilience, and Recovery for Everyone," https://www.dshs.state.tx.us/mhsa/trr/ (accessed April 2, 2015).

12. For an overview of this terminology and its implications, see the introduction to Geoffrey Nelson, Bret Kloos, and José Ornelas, eds., *Community Psychology and Community Mental Health: Towards Transformative Change* (New York: Oxford University Press, 2014), 3–20.

13. Gerald N. Grob, *The Mad Among Us: A History of the Care of America's Mentally Ill* (New York: The Free Press, 1994), 23–54.

14. David J. Rothman, *The Discovery of the Asylum: Social Order and Disorder in the New Republic*, rev. ed. (New York: Aldine Transaction, 2002 [1971]), 131–32.

15. Ibid., 236–65.

16. Rothman, *Conscience and Convenience: The Asylum and Its Alternatives in Progressive America*, rev. ed. (New York: Aldine de Gruyter, 2002 [1980]), 324–76.

17. Sarah C. Sitton, *Life at the Texas State Lunatic Asylum, 1857–1997* (College Station: Texas A&M University Press, 1999), 5.

Chapter 1

1. Text of Homer Rainey remarks, February 11, 1941, Box MAI9-U25, Hogg Foundation for Mental Health Records, Dolph Briscoe Center for American History, University of Texas at Austin (hereafter Hogg Foundation Papers). A similar quote appears in Kate Sayen Kirkland, *The Hogg Family and Houston: Philanthropy and the Civic Ideal* (Austin: University of Texas Press, 2009), 114–15.

2. Mary L. Praither Darden to Ima Hogg, July 26, 1939, Box 4W239, Ima Hogg Papers, 1824–1977, Dolph Briscoe Center for American History, University of Texas at Austin (hereafter Ima Hogg Papers).

3. Leopold L. Meyer to Ima Hogg, undated (c. 1939), Box 4W239, Ima Hogg Papers.

4. Minnie Fisher Cunningham to Ima Hogg, August 1, 1939; H.T. Manuel to Ima Hogg, August 18, 1939, Box 4W239, Ima Hogg Papers.

5. Henry C. Leach, President, The American-Scandinavian Foundation of New York, to Homer Rainey, August 8, 1939; Dorothy Gebauer, Dean of Women, University of Texas, to Homer Rainey, August 18, 1939; News Editor, *Journal of the American Medical Association*, to Homer Rainey, August 26, 1939; Evelyn M. Carrington, Texas Society for Mental Hygiene, to Homer Rainey, August 12, 1939; Dr. Minnie L. Maffett, MD, President, National Federation of Business and Professional Women's Clubs, to Homer Rainey, July 25, 1940; Elsie B. Jordt, Chair, San Antonio Branch of the American Association of University Women, Mental Hygiene Committee, to Homer Rainey, July 25, 1940. University of Texas President's Office Records, 1907–68, Dolph Briscoe Center for American History, University of Texas at Austin (hereafter President's Office Records).

6. Dr. H.D. White, MD, to Homer Rainey, July 31, 1939; J.A. Nelson to Homer Rainey, July 28, 1939; Blanche Carrier, Assistant Professor of Education, Northwestern University, to Homer Rainey, July 31, 1939; John M. Fletcher, professor emeritus of psychology, Tulane

University, to Homer Rainey, August 1, 1939, Box VF 18/D.b., President's Office Records.

7. William H. Jones, Dean, Tillotson College, to Homer Rainey, February 7, 1940; Homer Rainey to William H. Jones, February 10, 1940; Mortelia Womack to Homer Rainey, February 9, 1940; Homer Rainey to Mortelia Womack, February 14, 1940, Box VF 18/D.b., President's Office Records.

8. E.J. Cummins, President, El Paso Board of Education, to Homer Rainey, July 29, 1940; Prof. William T. Stanton, Mary Hardin-Baylor College, to Homer Rainey, July 31, 1940, Box VF 18/D.b., President's Office Records.

9. Elizabeth Moore to Homer Rainey, July 19, 1940, Box VF 18/D.b., President's Office Records.

10. Kirkland, *The Hogg Family and Houston*, 17.

11. Kirkland, *The Hogg Family and Houston*, 19; pages 14–29 offer a definitive family portrait and explore Ima's role in shaping the family's history in more depth; see also Greta Anderson, "Ima Hogg: Patroness of Texas," in *More Than Petticoats: Remarkable Texas Women* (Guilford, CT: Globe Pequot Press, 2002), 63–72; Louise Iscoe, *Ima Hogg: First Lady of Texas* (Austin, TX: Hogg Foundation for Mental Health, 1976); Gwendolyn Cone Neeley, *Miss Ima and the Hogg Family* (Dallas: Hendrick-Long, 1992); *Handbook of Texas Online*, s.v. "Hogg, Ima" http://www.tsha.utexas.edu/handbook/online/articles/HH/fho16.html (accessed July 13, 2005). For more on James Hogg, see Robert Cotner, *James Stephen Hogg, A Biography* (Austin: University of Texas Press, 1959). On Will C. Hogg, see John Avery Lomax, *Will Hogg, Texan* (Austin, TX: Hogg Foundation for Mental Health, 1956 [1940]).

12. Neeley, *Miss Ima and the Hogg Family*, 24. The Hogg family library included several books on mental health and illness, including Henry Maudsley, *Responsibility in Mental Disease* (New York: Appleton, 1878); William B. Carpenter, *Principles of Mental Physiology* (New York: Appleton, 1881); and Hugo Munsterberg, *Psychology and Life* (Boston: Houghton Mifflin, 1898). The entire list can be found in *Dedication Program, Will C. Hogg Building* (Austin, TX: Hogg Foundation for Mental Health, 1968).

13. Anderson, *More Than Petticoats*, 66.

14. "Robert L. Sutherland Interview with Miss Ima Hogg," August 24, 1970, Box MAI9-U25, Hogg Foundation Papers.

15. Virginia Bernhard, ed., *The Hoggs of Texas: Letters and Memoirs from an Extraordinary Family, 1887–1906* (Denton: Texas State Historical Association, 2013), 7.

16. Bernhard, *The Hoggs of Texas*, 206.

17. Neeley, *Miss Ima and the Hogg Family*, 32.

18. For more extended discussions, see Gerald N. Grob, *Mental Illness and American Society, 1875–1940* (Princeton, NJ: Princeton University Press, 1983), and David J. Rothman, *Conscience and Convenience: The Asylum and Its Alternatives in Progressive America*, 2d ed. (New York: Aldine de Gruyter, 2002).

19. "Conversation between Dr. Robert L. Sutherland and Miss Ima Hogg," May 10 and 13, 1967, p. 13, Box MAI9-U25, Hogg Foundation Records.

20. Kirkland, *The Hogg Family and Houston*, 29–30; Anderson, *More Than Petticoats*, 66.

21. Ibid.; see also "Transcription of Meeting at Miss Hogg's Home," March 8, 1962, pp. 2–3, Box MAI9-U25, Hogg Foundation Records.

22. Kirkland, *The Hogg Family and Houston*, 28–29.

23. Clifford W. Beers, *A Mind That Found Itself: An Autobiography* (Garden City, NY: Doubleday, 1948 [1908]), 255–380. Gerald N. Grob, *From Asylum to Community: Mental Health Policy in Modern America* (Princeton, NJ: Princeton University Press, 1991), 17–19.

24. "Texas Association for Mental Health, A Brief History," September 1973.

25. Kathleen W. Jones, *Taming the Troublesome Child: American Families, Child Guidance, and the Limits of Psychiatric Authority* (Cambridge, MA: Harvard University Press, 1999). Other book-length studies of child guidance include Margo Horn, *Before It's Too Late: The Child Guidance Movement in the United States, 1922–1945* (Philadelphia: Temple University Press, 1989), and Theresa R. Richardson, *The Century of the Child: The Mental Hygiene Movement and Social Policy in the United States and Canada* (Albany, NY: State University of New York Press, 1989).

26. Kirkland, *The Hogg Family and Houston*, 101–2.

27. See especially Jones, *Taming the Troublesome Child*, 91–119.

28. The entire report is reproduced in Gerald N. Grob ed., *Public Policy and Mental Illness: Four Investigations, 1915–1939* (New York: Arno Press, 1980).

29. Kirkland, *The Hogg Family and Houston*, 100; a full discussion of the national philanthropy movement can be found on 98–100.

30. Ibid., 102–5.

31. Fundraising letters, May 12, 1930; November 11, 1930; June 25, 1931; April 25, 1933, Box 4W235, Ima Hogg Papers.

32. *Annual Report of the Houston Child Guidance Clinic, 1931*, Ima Hogg Papers.

33. Kirkland, *The Hogg Family and Houston*, 106.

34. Neeley, *Miss Ima and the Hogg Family*, 71–72. See also Kirkland, *The Hogg Family and Houston*, 111–12.

35. Kirkland, *The Hogg Family and Houston*, 88–97.

36. Last Will and Testament of Will C. Hogg, March 7, 1928, Box 3B122, Ima Hogg Papers.

37. Neeley, *Miss Ima and the Hogg Family*, 72.

38. Meeting Minutes, University of Texas Board of Regents, July 15, 1939. Will C. Hogg Memorial Fund Files, Board of Regents Minutes (1939–59), University of Texas System Archives (hereafter UT System Archives).

39. "Will Hogg's Gift to Texas U. Recalls Service to Houston," *Houston Post*, July 21, 1939, p. 1

40. J.W. Calhoun to Homer Rainey, June 29, 1940; Calhoun to K.H. Aynesworth, July 15, 1940., Box VF18/D.b., President's Office Records.

41. "Memorandum Concerning the Purpose and General Policies of the Hogg Foundation," attachment, Robert L. Sutherland to Homer Rainey, September 19, 1940. A more public version of this connection appeared in a newspaper article describing a series of lectures Sutherland gave at Texas Tech University: "The educational lectureship and the mental hygiene objectives of the Hogg Foundation are not unrelated. Increasingly, the mental hygienist is thinking of mental health in terms of the total adjustment of personality to the social as well as the physical world. Increasingly the modern educator is measuring his results by the effects of education upon the adjustment of individuals in society." In other words, "modern trends bring these two fields ever closer together." News clipping attached to Robert L. Sutherland to Homer Rainey, July 20, 1942, President's Office Records.

42. Robert L. Sutherland to Homer Rainey, November 26, 1940, is the earliest dated correspondence written on letterhead; President's Office Records.

43. Robert L. Sutherland, "To Texans Interested in Public Education and Mental Hygiene," February 3, 1941, President's Office Records.

44. Robert L. Sutherland to Homer Rainey, October 11, 1940, President's Office Records.

45. Robert L. Sutherland to Mike Hogg, August 11, 1941, President's Office Records.

46. Robert L. Sutherland to Homer Rainey, March 16, 1942, President's Office Records.

47. Robert L. Sutherland to Homer Rainey, March 30 and April 3, 1942; Scott Gaines to Homer Rainey, April 17, 1942, President's Office Records.

48. Ima Hogg to Robert L. Sutherland, September 3, 1942, Ima Hogg Papers.

49. "President's Report on the Hogg Foundation," Meeting Minutes, University of Texas Board of Regents, October 23, 1942, UT System Archives.

50. "Report of Special Committee on Hogg Will," Meeting Minutes, University of Texas Board of Regents, January 8, 1943, UT System Archives.

51. "Hogg Foundation Program and Budget," lists the first budget at $32,103.96. Meeting Minutes, University of Texas Board of Regents, November 2, 1940, UT System Archives.

52. Meeting Minutes, University of Texas Board of Regents, July 15, 1939, UT System Archives.

53. Ima Hogg to Homer Rainey, September 16, 1939; Homer Rainey to Adolph Meyer, December 21, 1939; Homer Rainey to Daniel Prescott, December 21, 1939; Homer Rainey to George Stevenson, December 21, 1939; Adolph Meyer to Homer Rainey, December 28, 1939, Box VF 18/D.b., President's Office Papers.

54. Adolph Meyer to Ima Hogg, February 14, 1940, Box 4W239, Ima Hogg Papers.

55. Daniel Prescott to Homer Rainey, February 8, 1940, Box VF 18/D.b. President's Office Papers.

56. George Stevenson to Ima Hogg, December 14, 1940, Box 4W239, Ima Hogg Papers.

57. "Instructions to the Director from the Advisory Committee Which Met in Spring 1940," undated, Box MAI9-U23; Meeting Minutes, Committee on Mental Hygiene, January 30, 1940, Box MAI9-U25, Hogg Foundation Papers.

58. Memorandum, Robert L. Sutherland to Homer Rainey, "Special Policies Which Will Govern the Foundation During the Year 1940–1941," September 19, 1940, Box VF 5/E.b., President's Office Papers.

59. Evelyn M. Carrington to Homer Rainey, February 13, 1940, Box VF 18/E.b., President's Office Papers.

60. Homer Rainey to Ima Hogg, February 13, 1940, Box VF 18/E.b., President's Office Papers.

61. George Stevenson to Homer Rainey, February 7, 1940. President's Office Papers.

62. Homer Rainey to Ima Hogg, June 21, 1940, Box VF 18/E.b., President's Office Papers.

63. Homer Rainey to Robert Sutherland, March 25, 1940, Box MAI9-U14, Hogg Foundation Papers.

64. Quote from Robert Sutherland to Homer Rainey, June 17, 1940; the dialogue and negotiation is further documented in the following letters: Robert Sutherland to Homer Rainey, May 13, 1940; Homer Rainey to Robert Sutherland, May 15, 1940; Robert Sutherland to Homer Rainey, May 24, 1940; Robert Sutherland to Homer Rainey, June 3, 1940; Robert Sutherland to Homer Rainey, June 11, 1940; Homer Rainey to Robert Sutherland, June 15, 1940; Homer Rainey to Robert Sutherland, June 19, 1940, Box VF 18/E.b., President's Office Papers.

65. Homer P. Rainey, "A Personal Reminiscence," *The Hogg Foundation for Mental Health: The First Three Decades* (Austin: University of Texas, 1970), 3–5.

66. For short profiles of Robert Sutherland, see Kirkland, *The Hogg Family and Houston*, 115–16; Mary L. Kelley, *The Foundations of Texas Philanthropy* (College Station: Texas A&M University Press, 2004), 72–73; *Handbook of Texas Online*, s.v. "Sutherland, Robert Lee," http://www.tsha.utexas.edu/handbook/online/articles/SS/fsu15.html (accessed June 15, 2005); and Robert Sutherland, "An Analysis of Negro Churches in Chicago," unpublished PhD thesis (University of Chicago, 1930).

67. Key documents describing this project include Robert L. Sutherland, "Negro Youth: A Review of the Problems, Summary of Research, and a Recommended Program" (October

1937); Robert L. Sutherland, "A Proposed Study of Negro Youth Recommended to the American Youth Commission" (undated, c. winter 1937–38); Minutes, First Meeting of the Advisory Committee on the Negro Project, Washington, D.C., January 8, 1938. Sutherland Papers.

68. E. Franklin Frazier, *Negro Youth at the Crossways: Their Personality Development in the Middle States* (Washington, DC: American Council on Education, 1940); Allison Davis and John Dollard, *Children of Bondage: The Personality Development of Negro Youth in the Urban South* (Washington, DC: American Council on Education, 1940); and Charles S. Johnson, *Growing Up in the Black Belt: Negro Youth in the Rural South* (Washington, DC: American Council on Education, 1941).

69. Sutherland, *Color, Class, and Personality*, xv.

70. Author interview with Wayne Holtzman, November 12, 2013.

71. Robert Sutherland to F. Leland, November 12, 1941; "In Memoriam: Robert Lee Sutherland." Box MAI9-U14, Hogg Foundation Papers.

72. Robert Sutherland, "Relation Between Eschatology and Jesus' Ethics," unpublished MA thesis, Oberlin College, August 1927.

73. Author interview with Ira and Louise Iscoe, December 5, 2013.

Chapter 2

1. Lester Hamilton, "Palestine, TX (Anderson County)," *Handbook of Texas Online* (Denton: Texas State Historical Association), http://www.tshaonline.org/handbook/online/articles/hep01 (accessed July 22, 2014). On racial mores of the state at the time, see also Randolph B. Campbell, *Gone to Texas: A History of the Lone Star State* (New York: Oxford University Press, 2003), 419–29.

2. Joseph Howard Lumpkin, "Group Counseling and the Learning of Teacher Roles," unpublished PhD dissertation, University of Texas at Austin, 1954.

3. Joseph H. (Tony) Lumpkin to Robert L. Sutherland, September 6, 1952, Box MAI9-U28. Hogg Foundation Papers.

4. Lumpkin to Sutherland, February 6, 1952, and December 15, 1952, Box MAI9-U28. Hogg Foundation Papers.

5. *The Hogg Foundation Reports: A Summary of Three Years Work, A Forecast of Next Steps* (Austin: University of Texas, February 1944).

6. Ibid.

7. Unless otherwise noted, the following draws on Program Booklet, Bernice Milburn Moore Memorial Convocation, Hogg Foundation for Mental Health, June 17, 1993. Biographical Vertical File, "Moore, Bernice Milburn," Briscoe Center for American History, University of Texas at Austin.

8. Quote from Bernice Milburn Moore, "Biographical Statement, April 18, 1939, 1:45 p.m., in a mad rush," Biographical Vertical File, "Moore, Bernice Milburn;" also draws on author interview with Wayne Holtzman, November 12, 2013.

9. "New Type of Circuit Rider on Texas Program," *DeLeon Free Press*, undated clipping, c. January 1948, Box MAI9-U113–124, Hogg Foundation Papers.

10. "A Texas Resource: The Hogg Foundation for Mental Health," pamphlet, undated (c. 1973), Hogg Foundation for Mental Health vertical file, Briscoe Center for American History, University of Texas at Austin.

11. Author interview with Wayne Holtzman, November 12, 2013.

12. Unless otherwise noted, the following discussion draws on Gerald N. Grob, *From*

Asylum to Community: Mental Health Policy in Modern America (Princeton, NJ: Princeton University Press, 1991), 5–23; Gerald N. Grob, *The Mad Among Us: A History of the Care of America's Mentally Ill* (New York: The Free Press, 1994), 191–221; and Ellen Herman, *The Romance of American Psychology: Political Culture in the Age of Experts* (Berkeley: University of California Press, 1995), 48–123.

13. Harry C. Solomon and P.I. Yakovlev eds., *Manual of Military Neuropsychiatry* (Philadelphia: Saunders, 1944), 539, quoted in Grob, *From Asylum to Community*, 16.

14. Char Miller and David R. Johnson, "The Rise of Urban Texas," in Char Miller and Heywood T. Sanders, eds., *Urban Texas: Politics and Development* (College Station: Texas A&M University Press, 1990), 3–32; see also Ralph A. Wooster, "Over Here: Texans on the Home Front," in John W. Storey and Mary L. Kelley, eds., *Twentieth Century Texas: A Social and Cultural History* (Denton: University of North Texas Press, 2008), 164–195; and Campbell, *Gone to Texas*, 396–405.

15. Herman, *The Romance of American Psychology*, 238.

16. Grob, *From Asylum to Community*, 48, 90–91.

17. *The Hogg Foundation Reports*, 21–22. Beulah Temple Wild, "An Aid to Psychiatrists at Induction Stations," report attached to Robert L. Sutherland to J. Alton Burdine, October 1, 1943, Box VF5/E.b, President's Office Records.

18. "Mental Hygiene and Military Service," undated, c. August 1945, Box MAI9-U15, Hogg Foundation Papers.

19. Colonel Paul Wakefield to Robert L. Sutherland, October 15, 1943, Box MAI9-U15, Hogg Foundation Papers.

20. Robert L. Sutherland to Brigadier General William Lee Hart, August 4, 1945, Box MAI9-U15, Hogg Foundation Papers.

21. "Mental Hygiene and Military Service," pamphlet, March 1943, Box 4W235, Ima Hogg Papers; Rollo May, "Suggestions to the Counselor," pamphlet reprinted from the General Commission on Army and Navy Chaplains, undated, c. 1943, Box VF 11/E.a, President's Office Papers.

22. "Mental Growth Aids Happiness," *Daily Texan*, May 24, 1944.

23. "Child Who Knows He's Loved Isn't As Naughty," *El Paso Times*, April 4, 1941.

24. *The Hogg Foundation Reports*; "Mental Hygiene and Military Service," Hogg Foundation Papers.

25. "Dr. Sutherland to Give Suggestions to Combat Hysteria and War Nerves," *Austin Statesman*, April 6, 1942.

26. "Don't Let George Do It All: UT Scientist Tells How You Can Conquer 'War Nerves,'" *Austin Statesman*, April 9, 1942.

27. Ibid.

28. "Dr. Sutherland to Give Suggestions," supra note 20.

29. "Dr. Sutherland Talks Tonight on Personnel," *Beaumont Journal*, June 2, 1943.

30. "Speaker Declares Schools Must Make Readjustments to Meet War-Time Needs of Students," *Corsicana Sun*, May 1, 1942; "In-Service Training Courses for Teachers," 1944–45, Box 4W235, Ima Hogg Papers.

31. "Women in War Theme of Talks," *Amarillo News-Globe*, May 2, 1943.

32. "Dr. Bernice Moore Addresses P-T-A," *Rockdale Reporter*, May 13, 1943.

33. "WAC Gives Boost to Women's Equal Status," *Austin American*, October 11, 1943; see also "Dr. Moore Addresses Groups, Commends Correct Mental Stability Attitudes," *South Texan*, October 16, 1943.

34. Program Booklet, "Guidance for Youth in a World at War: An Institute for Teachers, Counselors, Group Workers, Service Club Members, and Parents," October 26–November 6, 1942, Box VF 11/E.a, President's Office Papers.

35. Program Booklet, "Adult Education, How to Get the Job Done," Third Annual Southwest Regional Conference on Adult Education, March 16–18, 1942, Stephen F. Austin Hotel, Austin, Texas, Box VF 11/E.a, President's Office Papers.

36. "Dr. Sutherland Addresses Child Welfare Conference," *Houston Chronicle*, January 26, 1944.

37. Grace Palladino, *Teenagers: An American History* (New York: Basic Books, 1998), 80–95. See also Kelly Schrum, *Some Wore Bobby Sox: The Emergence of Teenage Girls' Culture, 1920–1945* (New York: Palgrave Macmillan, 2004), 119; and William M. Tuttle, Jr., *Daddy's Gone to War: The Second World War in the Lives of America's Children* (New York: Oxford University Press, 1993), esp. 30–90. On teen canteens in Texas, see William S. Bush, *Who Gets a Childhood? Race and Juvenile Justice in Twentieth Century Texas* (Athens: University of Georgia Press, 2010), 51–52.

38. Lois Sager, "Preventing Wartime Delinquency," March 1943 pamphlet, Box VF 11/E.a, President's Office Papers.

39. Hogg Foundation mass mailing, February 1944, Box MAI9-U21, Hogg Foundation Papers.

40. Ibid.

41. Hogg Foundation mass mailing, October 4, 1943, Box VF 11/E.a, President's Office Papers.

42. "Mental Hygiene and Military Service," supra note 21; see also Robert L. Sutherland to Titus Harris, December 20, 1944; Sutherland to Thomas A.C. Rennie and Luther Woodward, December 20, 1944, Box MAI9-U15, Hogg Foundation Papers.

43. "Vets Procurement Advisory Board Planned," *Houston Press*, May 28, 1945.

44. "Self-Conscious Science and the Returning Veteran," lecture text attached to Robert L. Sutherland to Texas Social Welfare Association Representatives Who Attended the Inter-Agency Luncheon on December 7, 1944, Box 1991/016–58, Chairmen Lanning, Logan, Ashley, and Baker files, Texas State Board of Control Board members files, Archives and Information Services Division, Texas State Library and Archives Commission.

45. "Hogg Foundation to Co-operate in Post-War Readjustment," *Daily Texan*, March 9, 1944; "Hogg Brings Rehabilitator," *Daily Texan*, March 9, 1944; "Sutherland to Discuss Returning Soldiers," *Daily Texan*, March 23, 1944; "Veterans' View Told By Speaker: Men Back from Combat are Surprised at Attitude, Dr. Woodward Says," *Beaumont Journal*, December 12, 1944.

46. "Wartime Lessons for Educators," *Lubbock Avalanche*, June 15, 1945.

47. Ibid.

48. Robert L. Sutherland, *Essentials of a Community Mental Health Program: Tentative Guideposts for Community Planning* (Austin, TX: Hogg Foundation for Mental Hygiene, November 1945). See also R.L. Sutherland, "Society's Responsibility for Protecting the Mental Health of Children," *Texas State Journal of Medicine*, 37 (February 1942): 658–61.

49. Campbell, *Gone to Texas*, 411–12; Douglas Rossinow, *The Politics of Authenticity: Liberalism, Christianity, and the New Left in America* (New York: Columbia University Press, 1998), 23–28; Ronnie Dugger, *Our Invaded Universities: Form, Reform, and New Starts* (New York: Norton, 1974), 14–32.

50. Homer P. Rainey to Robert L. Sutherland, June 19, 1940, Box MAI9-U14, Hogg Foundation Papers.

51. Quote from Ima Hogg to Robert L. Sutherland, November 4, 1944; see also Ima Hogg to Homer Rainey, October 11, 1944; Homer Rainey to Ima Hogg, October 13, 1944; Mildred Rainey to Ima Hogg, December 2, 1944; Ima Hogg to State Senator Weaver Moore, January 27, 1945; Homer Rainey to Ima Hogg, February 5, 1945, Box 4W254, Ima Hogg Papers.

52. Burke Baker to Governor Coke Stevenson, November 21 and December 1, 1944; Sutherland to Ima Hogg, December 4, 1944; mass mailing of three Texas alumni in Austin, December 9, 1944, Box 4W254, Ima Hogg Papers.

53. Ima Hogg to Robert L. Sutherland, March 19, 1945; Ima Hogg to Dudley K. Woodward, March 19, 1945; Ima Hogg to Dudley K. Woodward, April 30, 1945, Box 4W254, Ima Hogg Papers.

54. "Endowed Hogg Foundation Service Vital," *Dallas Morning News*, January 1, 1943; see also "Clearing House for Community Problems Urged," *Galveston News*, November 9, 1943; "Dr. Overton Will Lecture October 20–22; Hogg Foundation and Committee Will Sponsor Appearances," *Beaumont Journal*, October 14, 1943.

55. Thomas B. Blackwell to Robert L. Sutherland, May 17, 1949, Box MAI9-U28, Hogg Foundation Papers.

56. "Family Life Conference Report," undated, c. 1949, Box MAI9-U28, Hogg Foundation Papers.

57. Edith Rockwood and Augusta J. Street, *Social Protective Work of Public Agencies, With Special Emphasis on the Policewoman* (Washington, DC: League of Women Voters, August 1932).

58. Augusta J. Street, "Report from Sabine School District, Gladewater, TX," March 21–22, 1949, Box MAI9-U28, Hogg Foundation Papers.

59. William R. Hunt, "MATADOR, TX," *Handbook of Texas Online*, http://www.tshaonline.org/handbook/online/articles/hjm07 (accessed August 7, 2014).

60. Augusta J. Street, "Report from Matador, TX," April 8, 1949, Box MAI9-U28, Hogg Foundation Papers.

61. Ibid.

62. Stephen L. Hardin, "Collegeport, TX," *Handbook of Texas Online*, http://www.tsha online.org/handbook/online/articles/hrc79 (accessed August 7, 2014).

63. Augusta J. Street, "Report from Collegeport," April 18, 1948, Box MAI9-U28, Hogg Foundation Papers.

64. Augusta J. Street, "Report from Grandfalls, Texas," March 28, 1951, Box MAI9-U28, Hogg Foundation Papers.

65. Augusta J. Street, "Report from Lubbock, Texas," April 6–7, 1949, Box MAI9-U28, Hogg Foundation Papers.

66. Ibid.

67. Postwar marriage data and mores are discussed in Elaine Tyler May, *Homeward Bound: American Families in the Cold War Era* (New York: Basic Books, 1988), 3–15; and Beth L. Bailey, *From Front Porch to Back Seat: Courtship in Twentieth Century America* (Baltimore, MD: Johns Hopkins University Press, 1989), 47–56.

68. Susan K. Cahn, *Sexual Reckonings: Southern Girls in a Troubling Age* (Cambridge, MA: Harvard University Press, 2007), 5.

69. Augusta J. Street, "Report from Alvin, Texas," March 23, 1948, Box MAI9-U28, Hogg Foundation Papers.

70. Augusta J. Street, "Report from Henderson, Texas," March 25, 1949, Box MAI9-U28, Hogg Foundation Papers.

71. Augusta J. Street, "Report from Shamrock, Texas," April 7, 1952, Box MAI9-U28, Hogg Foundation Papers.

72. "Report from Henderson, Texas," supra note 70.

73. Augusta J. Street, "Report from Orange, Texas," March 12, 1951, Box MAI9-U28, Hogg Foundation Papers.

74. "Cunningham's School Counseling Program," *Paris News*, November 25, 1945.

75. Augusta J. Street, "Report from Cunningham, Texas," April 4, 1952, Box MAI9-U28, Hogg Foundation Papers.

76. Augusta J. Street, "Report from Menard, Texas," February 17, 1948, Box MAI9-U28, Hogg Foundation Papers.

77. Augusta J. Street, "Report from Bay City, Texas," April 17, 1948, Box MAI9-U28, Hogg Foundation Papers.

78. Augusta J. Street, "Report from Pearsall, Texas," February 19–20, 1948, Box MAI9-U28, Hogg Foundation Papers.

79. *An Idea Worth Fulfilling: History of the School of Social Work, 1950–1983* (Austin: University of Texas School of Social Work, 2010), 1–7.

80. "Schools in Texas for Social Work Declared Needed," *Houston Chronicle*, April 8, 1948.

81. "Social Work Described as Money-Saver," *Dallas Morning News*, May 3, 1941.

82. "In-Service Training Courses for Teachers," curriculum guides and course descriptions, 1944–45, Box 4W235, Ima Hogg Papers.

83. Robert L. Sutherland, *Essentials of a Community Mental Health Program: Tentative Guideposts for Community Planning* (Austin, TX: Hogg Foundation for Mental Hygiene, November 1945).

84. Elizabeth F. Gardner, "Annotated List of Lecturers and Consultants for the Hogg Foundation, 1941–1956." Box MAI9-U21, Hogg Foundation Papers.

85. Memo, Sutherland to Hogg Foundation advisors, September 29, 1953, Box 3M390, Sutherland Papers.

86. "Program of Community Activities for 1949–1950," West Side Community House, Inc., Box MAI9-U23, Hogg Foundation Papers.

87. Jesse J. Villereal, "Summary of Activities on Trip, January 18–21, 1950, Under Sponsorship of the Hogg Foundation, to Visit Local Programs in Speech and Hearing Therapy in the Houston-Beaumont-Galveston Area," February 8, 1950, Box MAI9-U23, Hogg Foundation Papers.

88. "Special School Problems Cited—50 Persons Hear Dr. Jesse J. Villareal of Texas University Speak," *Beaumont Enterprise*, January 21, 1950, news clipping; letter, Sadie Aaron to Robert Sutherland, April 17, 1944, Box MAI9-U23, Hogg Foundation Papers.

89. "Charter of the Woman's Foundation, Inc.," February 1942, Box MAI9-U31, Hogg Foundation Papers.

90. James M. Wood, "Unwanted Women," *Women's Home Companion* (May 1948), 38–40; Wood, "Let the Women In!" Clippings in Box MAI9-U31, Hogg Foundation Papers.

91. See May, *Homeward Bound*, 58–92.

92. Wood, "Let the Women In!" supra note 89.

93. "Charter of the Woman's Foundation, Inc.," supra note 89.

94. Untitled brochure, Woman's Foundation, Inc., March 1950, Box MAI9-U31, Hogg Foundation Papers.

95. Ibid.

96. Mark Odintz, "Slocum, TX," *Handbook of Texas Online*, http://www.tshaonline.org/handbook/online/articles/hls57 (accessed August 8, 2014).

97. Quote from E.R. Bills, "Town's 1910 Racial Strife A Nearly Forgotten Piece of Texas' Past," *Austin American-Statesman*, February 23, 2013; see also Bills, *The 1910 Slocum Massacre: An Act of Genocide in East Texas* (Charleston, SC: The History Press, 2014).

98. Ibid. See H.R. 865, Acknowledging the Slocum massacre of 1910, 82nd sess., 2011, http://www.legis.state.tx.us/.

99. "Development of Woman's Foundation-Hogg Foundation Project in Slocum," January 13, 1947, Box MAI9-U31, Hogg Foundation Papers.

100. Slocum Rural Family Life Project, Minutes of Meetings Various Committees, December 14, 1946–January 28, 1947 (received February 11, 1947), Box MAI9-U31, Hogg Foundation Papers.

101. Ernest E. Neal, Consultant, Monthly Report of Family Life and Educational Council, Union Hope School, January 19, 1947, Box MAI9-U31, Hogg Foundation Papers.

102. J.C. McAdams, consultant report, October 1947, Box MAI9-U31, Hogg Foundation Papers.

103. Consultant report, Union Hope School, March 10, 1947, Box MAI9-U31, Hogg Foundation Papers.

104. "Memo on the Slocum, Texas Family Life Study," undated, c. February 1947, Box MAI9-U31, Hogg Foundation Papers.

105. Ernest E. Neal to Robert L. Sutherland, February 11, 1971, Box MAI9-U14, Hogg Foundation Papers.

106. Ernest E. Neal, consultant, "Monthly Report of Family Life and Educational Council Union Hope School," May 1947, Box MAI9-U31, Hogg Foundation Papers.

107. Ernest E. Neal, consultant, "Monthly Report of Family Life and Educational Council, Union Hope School," August 1947, Box MAI9-U31, Hogg Foundation Papers.

108. Ernest E. Neal to Dora Hassell, December 13, 1947, Box MAI9-U31, Hogg Foundation Papers.

109. Ernest E. Neal, consultant, "Monthly Report of Family Life and Educational Council Union Hope School," July 1947, Box MAI9-U31, Hogg Foundation Papers.

110. Dora Hassell to Ernest E. Neal, May 24, 1947; Ernest E. Neal to Robert L. Sutherland, May 29, 1947, Box MAI9-U31, Hogg Foundation Papers.

111. The full internal note reads as follows: "Letters about the Negro scholarships should be saved and kept together because they illustrate an interesting problem that arose. It appears to be rooted in some rather definite attitudes of prejudice on the part of Mrs. Hassell, but I am not sure." Robert L. Sutherland, file note, Slocum Rural Family Life Project folder, undated, c. May 1947, Box MAI9-U31, Hogg Foundation Papers.

112. Robert L. Sutherland to Lloyd Allan Cook, May 4, 1948, Box MAI9-U31, Hogg Foundation Papers.

113. Dora Hassell to Robert L. Sutherland, April 24, 1948, Box MAI9-U31, Hogg Foundation Papers.

114. Robert L. Sutherland to Lillian Peek, May 3, 1948, Box MAI9-U31, Hogg Foundation Papers.

115. "Evidence of Progress Made in Slocum During the Period Covered by the Study," undated, c. spring 1948, Box MAI9-U31, Hogg Foundation Papers.

Chapter 3

1. J.P. Porter, "Mental Hospitals Have No Alumni to Endow Them—Only the People," *Daily Texan*, January 11, 1949. "Hogg Foundation for Mental Health" Vertical File, Briscoe Center for American History, University of Texas at Austin.

2. Ibid.

3. "Houston Group to Hear Crusading U. of T. Student," *Houston Press*, February 18, 1949.

4. Chris Whitcraft, "A Revolution Brews in Mental Health Care," *Austin American-Statesman*, February 5, 1956. The history of mental health reforms in the 1950s is summarized in Sitton, *Life at the Texas State Lunatic Asylum*, 132–42; and Mikel Jean Fisher Brightman, "An Historical Survey of the State of Texas' Efforts to Aid the Mentally Ill and the Mentally Retarded," unpublished MA thesis, University of Texas, 1971, 13–32. For more on Connally, see James Reston Jr., *The Lone Star: The Life of John Connally* (New York: Harper Collins, 1989) and, more recently, Carlos Kevin Blanton, "The Campus and the Capitol: John B. Connally and the Struggle Over Texas Higher Education Policy, 1950–1970," *Southwestern Historical Quarterly*, 108.4 (April 2005): 468–97.

5. Gerald N. Grob, *The Mad Among Us: A History of the Care of America's Mentally Ill* (New York: The Free Press, 1994), 202–3. See also Richard G. Frank, *Better But Not Well: Mental Health Policy in the United States Since 1950* (Baltimore, MD: Johns Hopkins University Press, 2006), 1–7.

6. Grob, *The Mad Among Us*, 203.

7. Albert Deutsch, *The Shame of the States* (New York: Harcourt, Brace, and Co., 1948), 31.

8. Ibid., 38–39.

9. Ibid.; Grob, *The Mad Among Us*, 203–4.

10. Grob, *The Mad Among Us*, 204–6.

11. "Mental Health," *Handbook of Texas Online*, http://www.tshaonline.org/handbook/online/articles/smmun (accessed October 23, 2013).

12. Samuel W. Hamilton, *Survey of State Mental Institutions of Texas* (Austin: Texas State Board of Control, 1943).

13. Weaver H. Baker to Robert L. Sutherland, January 12, 1942, and January 21, 1942, Box 1991/016–58, Chairmen Lanning, Logan, Ashley, and Baker files, Texas State Board of Control Board members files, Archives and Information Services Division, Texas State Library and Archives Commission (hereafter TSBC Members Files).

14. Ibid.

15. Sutherland to Baker, January 16, 1943; Baker to Sutherland, January 18, 1943; Sutherland to Baker, February 19, 1943; Baker to Sutherland, February 20, 1943; Sutherland to Baker, February 26, 1943; Sutherland to Baker, September 4, 1943; Baker to Sutherland, September 13, 1943; Sutherland to Baker, September 17, 1943; Baker to Sutherland, November 27, 1944, TSBC Members Files.

16. Program Booklet, Texas Society for Mental Hygiene Annual Conference, Dallas, Texas, March 4–5, 1943, TSBC Members Files.

17. Sutherland to Baker, April 29, 1943; Baker to Sutherland, May 1, 1943, TSBC Members Files.

18. Ibid; the seminar is also discussed in Sutherland to Baker, June 7, 1943; Baker to Sutherland, June 8, 1943; quote from undated flyer, "The Hogg Foundation Presents Russell L. Dicks," TSBC Members Files.

19. C. Ellis Nelson and Milton A. Maxwell, "Report on the Vesper Project at the Austin

State Hospital," July 1943; Sutherland to Baker, November 20, 1943; Baker to Sutherland, November 22, 1943; Charles Castner to Baker, November 26, 1943, TSBC Members Files.

20. The summary and quotes that follow draw from Samuel W. Hamilton, "Life in Our Mental Hospitals: Its Meaning for the Individual," *Mental Hygiene*, 27.1 (January 1943): 3–9.

21. Letter to all state hospital superintendents, Robert L. Sutherland and Weaver H. Baker, June 4, 1943, TSBC Members Files.

22. Ibid.

23. Dr. William Thomas, Superintendent, Terrell Hills State Hospital, to Robert L. Sutherland, Weaver H. Baker, and Charles Castner, June 9, 1943, TSBC Members Files.

24. *Texas Trends: Official Publication of the Texas Society for Mental Hygiene* 1.2 (February 1944); *Texas Eleemosynary Trends: The Work of Our State Schools and Hospitals* 1.1 (February 1944), TSBC Members Files.

25. Charles W. Castner, "State Mental Hospitals in Texas," *Texas Trends*, 1.2 (February 1944): 9–12.

26. A.T. Hanretta, "Present and Potential Community Services of Texas State Hospitals," *Texas Trends*, 1.2 (February 1944): 21–24.

27. Texas State Board of Control, Memo to Heads of State Institutions, April 14, 1944, TSBC Members Files.

28. Ibid.

29. Baker to Sutherland, October 18, 1944; Sutherland to Baker, November 8, 1944, TSBC Members Files.

30. For example, the following year, the Foundation purchased one hundred subscriptions to *The Attendant*, a newsletter published by the mental hygiene program of the Civilian Public Service, a wartime agency. Sutherland to Baker, July 17, 1945; Baker to Sutherland, July 19, 1945; "A Patient's-Eye View of Nurses and Attendants," *The Attendant*, 2.7 (July 1945), TSBC Members Files.

31. Charles W. Castner to Sutherland, October 1, 1945, TSBC Members Files.

32. Sutherland to Baker, November 2, 1944; Sutherland to Baker, June 29, 1945; Baker to Sutherland, June 30, 1945, TSBC Members Files.

33. Sutherland to Baker, March 19, 1945; Baker to Sutherland, March 21, 1945, TSBC Members Files.

34. TSMH mass mailing to members from Elizabeth F. Gardner, TSMH Secretary, December 1945; Postcard, TSMH to Baker, April 25, 1946, TSBC Members Files.

35. "Weaver Baker Rites Are Held Here Wednesday," *Junction Eagle*, September 22, 1946.

36. All quotes in the following discussion draw on Jack R. Ewalt, "Public Care of the Mentally Ill in Texas," *Texas Trends*, 4.2 (January 1947): 7–14.

37. Ibid., 11–12.

38. Sutherland to Hall H. Logan, February 8, 1947; Logan to Sutherland, February 17, 1947, TSBC Members Files.

39. Logan to Sutherland, February 17, 1947, TSBC Members Files.

40. Report of the Legislative Committee on Eleemosynary and Reformatory Institutions, April 23, 1947, 3–6.

41. Ibid., 6–7.

42. Ibid., 9–10.

43. Ibid., 13.

44. S.B. 374, 50th Session, General and Special Laws of Texas, Legislative Reference Library.

45. Sutherland to Logan, April 22, 1947, TSBC Members Files.

46. Logan to Sutherland, April 30, 1947; Sutherland to Logan, May 1, 1947; Sutherland to Logan, May 5, 1947; Sutherland to Logan, May 30, 1947, TSBC Members Files.

47. John P. Porter to Sutherland, March 11, 1949, Box MAI9-U27, Hogg Foundation Papers.

48. "Agreement Between J.P. Porter and the Hogg Foundation," February 14, 1949, Box MAI9-U27, Hogg Foundation Papers. On funding, see "Student's Articles Win $100 Award," *Dallas Times Herald*, April 1, 1949.

49. J.P. Porter, "The Shame of Texas: State Has No Brag Coming on Mental Hospital Condition," *Austin American-Statesman*, March 20, 1949. Other articles in the series as follows: "3–21–49, "The Shame of Texas: Senile Patients Jammed into State Hospitals," *Austin American*, March 21, 1949; "The Shame of Texas: Mentally Ill Now Must Watch Others Get Shock Treatment," *Austin American*, March 22, 1949; "The Shame of Texas: State Hospital Offers Exhibit 'A' in Misery," *Austin American*, March 23, 1949; "The Shame of Texas: Unplanned, Tottering Hospital 'Just Grew,'" *Austin American*, March 24, 1949; "The Shame of Texas: Epileptic Hospital at Abilene Called Death Trap by Worker," *Austin American*, March 25, 1949; "The Shame of Texas: Worn-Out Rusk Penitentiary Serves as Mental Hospital," *Austin American*, March 26, 1949; "The Shame of Texas: State Hospital Life Spawns Violent Death," *Austin American*, March 27, 1949. Clippings of these articles from the *Dallas Morning News*, *Houston Post*, *Paris Daily News*, and *Abilene Reporter-News* are collected in Box MAI9-U113–124, Hogg Foundation Papers.

50. Ibid.

51. "The Shame of Texas: State Hospital Life Spawns Violent Death."

52. "Lawmakers Hear Plea for Welfare Laws," *Houston Post*, February 19, 1949; the eyewitness account comes from Helen Seymour to Sutherland, February 22, 1949, in which she also thanks Sutherland for sending Porter to speak at the panel; Box MAI9-U27, Hogg Foundation Papers.

53. Postcard, Sutherland to Logan, undated, c. February 1949; Sutherland to Logan, February 14, 1949; Sutherland to Logan, February 26, 1949, TSBC Members Files.

54. Sutherland to Logan, March 9, 1949; Logan to Sutherland, March 14, 1949; Sutherland to Logan, March 17, 1949, TSBC Members Files.

55. H.B. 1, 51st Session, 1949, *General and Special Laws of Texas*, reprinted in Board Policy Circulars of the Board of Texas State Hospitals and Special Schools (Vol. 1), August 1955, Box 2005/096–2, Minutes, Texas Board for Texas State Hospitals and Special Schools records. Archives and Information Services Division, Texas State Library and Archives Commission (hereafter Board Policy Circulars).

56. "Governor Shivers Will Support Amendment," *Bracketville News Mail Weekly*, September 25, 1949; "Texas to Vote Next Month on Constitution Changes," *Dublin Progress Weekly*, October 21, 1949; "'Lunacy' Panel To Be Broadcast." *Marshall News-Messenger*, October 30, 1949, Box MAI9-U111–112, Hogg Foundation Papers. "Amendments Defeated," *Austin Statesman*, undated, c. November 1949; Editorial, *McLean News*, November 17, 1949, Box MAI9-U113–124, Hogg Foundation Papers.

57. Albert D. Pattillo, Superintendent, Terrell State Hospital, to Robert L. Sutherland, September 8, 1949; Mrs. J.C. Clemons to Sutherland, October 8, 1949, Box MAI9-U27, Hogg Foundation Papers.

58. "Disgraceful Condition of State Mental Hospitals Is Exposed by Tour of Texas Newspapermen," *Bellville Times Weekly*, November 24, 1949; "Mental Institutions Over-Crowded, Staffs Overworked, Newsmen Find," *San Jacinto Times*, December 21, 1949; "Mental Hospi-

tals Badly Understaffed," *North Texas American*, January 5, 1950, Box MAI9-U111–112, Hogg Foundation Papers.

59. "State Mental Hospitals Far Below APA Standard," *Wichita Daily Times*, January 7, 1950, "Mentally Ill Care In State Called Worst In Nation, *Palestine Herald-Press*, January 14, 1950, and *Harlingen Valley Morning Star*, January 14, 1950, Box MAI9-U111–112, Hogg Foundation Papers.

60. James S. Mahon, State Chair, Jaycee Committee on Mental Health, "Mental Hygiene," mass mailing, June 13, 1949, Box MAI9-U27, Hogg Foundation Papers.

61. "Texas Legislators Will Face a Double Headed Program Tuesday," *Wichita Daily Times*, January 26, 1950; "Cigarettes Levy Now Draws Fire," *San Angelo Standard-Times*, January 28, 1950; "Texas Needs $25 Million in Hospital Funds: Painless Way to Raise Money in Election Year Is Legislators' Problem," *Baytown Sun Daily*, January 31, 1950.

62. *Report of the Board for Texas State Hospitals and Special Schools, From September 1, 1949 to December 1, 1950* (Austin: Texas Board for State Hospitals and Special Schools, 1950), 8–14.

63. Ibid.; see also "Million People Treated for Mental Illness," *Houston Press*, January 4, 1950.

64. "Institute Puts Texas 37th in Mental Health," *Fort Worth Star-Telegram*, January 22, 1950.

65. "Memorandum Concerning State Hospital Board," undated, c. January 1950; "Memorandum, Proposal of the Board of Texas State Hospitals and Special Schools to the Legislature," undated, c. January 1950, Box MAI9-U27, Hogg Foundation Papers. See also "APA Director Reports on Mental Hospitals," *Austin Statesman*, January 30, 1950.

66. Mass mailing, Jim Mahon, Chairman, Texas Jaycees Mental Health Committee, undated, c. fall 1949; mass mailing, Moyne L. Kelly, Executive Director, Board of Texas State Hospitals and Special Schools, undated, c. fall 1949, Box MAI9-U27, Hogg Foundation Papers.

67. "Legislature's Special Session Begins Today," *Big Spring Herald Daily*, January 31, 1950.

68. Allan Shivers, "Legislature Shows Interest in State Hospital Problems," *Austin Statesman*, February 16, 1950.

69. Boyce Campbell, Director, "Shock Treatment," script and notes, Austin, Texas, January 1950, Box MAI9-U27, Hogg Foundation Papers.

70. Ibid.

71. Joe Belden, "Texans Awake on Hospitals," *Waco Tribune Herald*, January 15, 1950; "Public Behind State Hospital Improvements," *Cuero Daily Record*, January 15, 1950.

72. "Texans Get Governor Shivers Told on How to Finance Hospitals," *Mineral Wells Index*, January 20, 1950.

73. TSMH mass mailing, undated, c. January 1950, Box MAI9-U27, Hogg Foundation Papers.

74. Report of the Meeting of the Citizens Committee on Mental Health, January 30, 1950, Box MAI9-U27, Hogg Foundation Papers.

75. Ibid.

76. Hogg Foundation mass mailing, undated, c. January 1950, Box MAI9-U27, Hogg Foundation Papers.

77. Allan Shivers to Robert L. Sutherland, February 4, 1950, Box MAI9-U27, Hogg Foundation Papers.

78. "Address by Honorable Allan Shivers, Governor," February 1, 1950, *Journal of the*

House of Representatives of the First Called Session of the Fifty-First Legislature of the State of Texas, January 31, 1950, pp. 11–15.

79. Ibid., 13.

80. Ibid., 14.

81. "Leaders Favor Hospital Plans," *Dallas Morning News*, February 1, 1950; "Governor Warns of Fire Hazards in Texas Hospitals," *Kilgore News Herald*, February 2, 1950.

82. *The Hogg Foundation Reports: Twelve Years of Mental Health Work in Texas* (Austin: University of Texas Press, 1953), 19–21.

83. Meeting Minutes, Texas Society for Crippled Children, April 11, 1950, Box VF5/E.b., UT President's Office Papers.

84. "Omnibus Tax Tops Revenue Proposal," *Austin American*, February 2, 1950; "Tax Hike Backers Win First Test," *Corpus Christi Times*; February 2, 1950; "Oil, Gas Men Agree to Tax as New Fund," *Edinburg Daily Review*, February 7, 1950; "Senate Votes 20 Million for Hospitals, Schools," *Hillsboro Evening Mirror*, February 8, 1950; "Texas House Finally Passes School, Hospital Money Bill," *Corsicana Sun*, February 10, 1950.

85. "Senator Receives Many Local Letters Urging Hospital Appropriations," *El Campo News*, February 17, 1950.

86. *Newsletter of the Board for Texas State Hospitals and Special Schools* 1.4 (August 1, 1950), Box MAI9-U27, Hogg Foundation Papers.

87. "Notes Taken at the Hearing on S.B. 278, March 12, 1951," attached to mass mailer, Texas Social and Legislative Conference, March 14, 1951; "Summary of Charges Against the State Hospital Board," undated, c. spring 1951, Box MAI9-U27, Hogg Foundation Papers.

88. "TB Committee Protests Return-to-Board Proposal," *Dallas Morning News*, March 1, 1951; "State Hospital Board," editorial, *Bryan Daily Eagle*, March 14, 1951; "Suspicious Move: Why Change Horses?" *Lubbock Morning Avalanche*, March 15, 1951; "Why Junk the State Hospital Board?" editorial, *Port Arthur News*, March 21, 1951; "Dual Hospital Control Sparks Senate Storm," *Dallas Daily Times Herald*, March 28, 1951.

89. "Committee Favors Abolishing Hospital, Special School Board," *Dallas Morning News*, March 13, 1951.

90. Ibid.

91. Memo, Leslie L. O'Connor, BTSHSS, to Robert L. Sutherland, August 31, 1950, Box MAI9-U27, Hogg Foundation Papers.

92. "Notes Taken at the Hearing," supra note 87.

93. Mass mailing, James Mahon to Texas Jaycees, undated, c. March 16, 1951, Box MAI9-U27, Hogg Foundation Papers.

94. Mass mailing, James Mahon to Texas Jaycees, March 29, 1951, Box MAI9-U27, Hogg Foundation Papers.

95. Mass mailing, Ozro T. Woods, Citizens Committee on Mental Health, March 30, 1951, Box MAI9-U27, Hogg Foundation Papers.

96. Hamilton Ford to Chancellor James Hart, April 7, 1951; Ford to Robert L. Sutherland, April 8, 1951, Box MAI9-U27, Hogg Foundation Papers.

97. This and all subsequent quotes draw from the following: Meeting Summary, "The Hogg Foundation for Mental Health, Its Relation to Public Agencies," July 9, 1951, Box MAI9-U25, Hogg Foundation Papers.

98. "Interview with Miss Hogg," November 21, 1961.

99. Author interview with Wayne Holtzman, November 21, 2013.

100. Biographical data sheet, undated; Carolyn Bengtson, "Outstanding Careerwoman," *Austin American*, January 22, 1966; Janet Wilson, "When a Caretaker Needs Care," May 2,

1999, *Austin American–Statesman.* "Bert Kruger Smith" Vertical File, Briscoe Center for American History

101. Nomination letter, Edith M. Stern to Mrs. Howard W. Blakeslee, September 25, 1960, Bert Kruger Smith Papers, Box 3A210–211, Briscoe Center for American History.

102. Author interview with Ira and Louise Iscoe, December 5, 2013.

103. Bert Kruger Smith, "Behind the Walls of Texas State Hospitals," undated news clippings, November 1952–February 1953, Box MAI9-U111–112, Hogg Foundation Papers.

104. "14-Point Care and Treatment Program," Board Policy Circular M-10, June 14, 1952, Board Policy Circulars. This circular is reproduced in "Facts Are Facts," Texas Society for Mental Hygiene pamphlet, undated, c. 1952, Box MAI9-U27, Hogg Foundation Papers.

105. "Organization and Functions of the Board of Texas State Hospitals and Special Schools," 1950, Board Policy Circulars.

106. Gerald N. Grob, *From Asylum to Community: Mental Health Policy in Modern America* (Princeton, NJ: Princeton University Press, 1991), 89–93.

107. Report of the Public Service Committee of the Texas Society for Mental Hygiene, March 3, 1952; Meeting Minutes, May 8, 1952; "Proposed Legislative Program," May 19, 1952; "Memo on 14-Point Program," June 6, 1952, Box MAI9-U27, Hogg Foundation Papers.

108. Robert L. Sutherland to Ozro Woods and Don Morris, March18, 1953, Box MAI9-U27, Hogg Foundation Papers.

109. Meeting Minutes, May 18, 1953, Box 1998/147–1. Minutes, Texas Board for Texas State Hospitals and Special Schools records. Archives and Information Services Division, Texas State Library and Archives Commission (hereafter BTSHSS Minutes).

110. Meeting Minutes, July 13 and September 9, 1953, BTSHSS Minutes.

111. Meeting Minutes, February 15 and March 15, 1954, BTSHSS Minutes.

112. Mass mailing, Hogg Foundation for Mental Health, April 13, 1954, Box MAI9-U27, Hogg Foundation Papers.

113. Meeting Minutes, April 13, 1954, BTSHSS Minutes.

114. Ibid; "Ideas Presented at April 13, 1954 Meeting of Sub-Committee to Advisory Committee," Box MAI9-U27, Hogg Foundation Papers.

115. "Groups Map Statewide Drive to Better Schools, Hospitals," *Austin Statesman*, April 14, 1954; "Hospitals Improved, But More Needed," *Austin American-Statesman*, September 3, 1954; "Panel to 'Advise' on State Hospitals," *Dallas Times Herald*, December 14, 1954.

116. Meeting Minutes, April 11 and June 13, 1955, BTSHSS Minutes.

117. Advisory Committee Meeting Notes with Governor Allan Shivers, June 22, 1954; other activities documented in Advisory Committee Minutes, Tour of San Antonio State Hospital, June 11, 1954; "An Intermediate Program for the Care and Training of Mentally Retarded Children and Adults in the State of Texas," November 1954; Aris A. Mallas Jr., project director, Texas Research League, to John W. Dudley, June 15, 1955; Memo, conference call with Robert L. Sutherland and Vernon McGee, Legislative Budget Board, undated, c. 1955, Box MAI9-U27, Hogg Foundation Papers.

118. Meeting Minutes, August 2, 1954, BTSHSS Minutes.

119. Meeting Minutes, September 20, 1954, BTSHSS Minutes.

120. Sutherland to Mrs. Lawrence Tarlton, BTSHSS member, May 25, 1954; Advisory Committee Meeting Notes, June 9, 1954; Ed Bridges to Sutherland, June 24, 1954; Sutherland to Bridges, October 1, 1954; Henry L. Hoskins to Sutherland, November 22, 1954; Sutherland to Hoskins, November 24, 1954, Box MAI9-U27, Hogg Foundation Papers.

121. Memo, Ed Bridges, BTSHSS Public Information Committee, to Sutherland, June 9, 1955, Box MAI9-U27, Hogg Foundation Papers.

122. The session's legislation was summarized in Bert Kruger Smith, *The Turning Key* [Pamphlet] (Austin, TX: Hogg Foundation for Mental Health, 1955).

123. Robert L. Sutherland to William Menninger, June 10, 1955, Box MAI9-U27, Hogg Foundation Papers.

124. Meeting Minutes, Advisory Committee, January 13 and March 28, 1956, Box MAI9-U27, Hogg Foundation Papers.

125. Robert L. Sutherland to Mary Butt, February 18, 1956, and March 16, 1956, Box MAI9-U27, Hogg Foundation Papers.

126. "Consultant's Report on Proposed Mental Health Program for the State of Texas," June 3, 1956, Box MAI9-U27, Hogg Foundation Papers.

127. Transcribed phone conference, Robert L. Sutherland, Wayne H. Holtzman, and Robert Felix, September 1956, Box MAI9-U27, Hogg Foundation Papers.

128. The following discussion draws on Bert Kruger Smith, dir., *In a Strange Land* (Austin, TX: Hogg Foundation for Mental Health, 1956); and, script and notes, Box MAI9-U111–112, Hogg Foundation Papers.

129. Texas Research League, "A Statement Concerning the Texas Mental Health Code Drafting Project," July 1955, Box MAI9-U27, Hogg Foundation Papers.

130. Millard Ruud to Dean Page Keeton, June 8, 1956, Box MAI9-U27, Hogg Foundation Papers.

131. Connally quoted in Chris Whitcraft, "A Revolution Brews in Mental Health Care," *Austin American-Statesman*, February 5, 1956.

132. Robert L. Sutherland to Senator Searcy Bracewell, May 3, 1955; Bracewell to Sutherland, May 16, 1955; Sutherland to Bracewell, May 23, 1955; Sutherland to Ima Hogg, May 23, 1955; Ima Hogg to Senator A. M. Aikin Jr., January 8, 1957, Box MAI9-U28, Hogg Foundation Papers.

133. "Outline of the Proposed Remarks of William C. Menninger, M.D.," undated; Menninger Foundation to Texas State Legislature, February 12, 1957, Box MAI9-U28, Hogg Foundation Papers.

134. "Expert Asks for Fair Shake for State's Mentally Ill," *Austin American-Statesman*, February 12, 1957; "Time to Buy Both Bricks and Brains," *Dallas Morning News*, February 15, 1957, Box MAI9-U28, Hogg Foundation Papers.

135. Section 2, H.B. 6, *General and Special Laws of Texas*, 55th Session, 1957.

136. Ibid; see also Millard H. Ruud, *Interpretation of the Mental Health Code*, 1st ed. (Austin: University of Texas Press, 1957).

137. "Mental Health Code Faces First Test," *Amarillo Globe-Times*, February 13, 1957; "Mental Health Group Urges Code Okay," *San Angelo Standard Times*, April 14, 1957; "New Mental Health Code," *Austin American-Statesman*, April 15, 1957.

Chapter 4

1. Elaine Tyler May, *Homeward Bound: American Families in the Cold War Era* (New York: Basic Books, 1988), 3–9, 26–27.

2. "Meet Mr. Pelican," undated mailer, c. 1947, Box MAI9-U21, Hogg Foundation Papers.

3. Ibid.

4. The following discussion draws on the Hogg Foundation pamphlet reprint of Loyd W. Rowland, "A Mental Health Project in Louisiana," *American Journal of Mental Deficiency*, 52.2 (October 1947); "Method of Using the Pierre the Pelican Materials: A Manual" (Loui-

siana Society for Mental Health, 1947); and, *The Pierre the Pelican Series*, 12 vols., undated, c. 1948, Box MAI9-U21, Hogg Foundation Papers.

5. Ibid.

6. Ibid.

7. May, *Homeward Bound*, 26.

8. Woman's Foundation, Inc., to Loyd W. Rowland, October 18, 1946; Loyd W. Rowland to Robert L. Sutherland, October 22, 1946, Box MAI9-U21, Hogg Foundation Papers.

9. Loyd W. Rowland, "A First Evaluation of the Pierre the Pelican Mental Health Pamphlets," in L.R. Rowland, ed., *The Louisiana Mental Health Studies*, Vol. 1 (New Orleans: Louisiana Society for Mental Health, November 1948).

10. *The Pierre the Pelican Series*, 12 vols. (undated, c. 1948); Box MAI9-U21, Hogg Foundation Papers.

11. Catherine Mackenzie, "The First Year," *New York Times Magazine*, February 29, 1948.

12. This section draws in part on Mary L. Kelley, *The Foundations of Texan Philanthropy* (College Station: Texas A&M University Press, 2005), 70–80. In 2014 the organization was renamed Philanthropy Southwest. See www.philanthropysouthwest.org (accessed September 24, 2014).

13. Kelley, *The Foundations of Texas Philanthropy*, 70–71, 91–95.

14. "The Conference of Southwest Foundations," undated, c. 1960, Box MAI9-U21, Hogg Foundation Papers.

15. Kelley, *The Foundations of Texas Philanthropy*, 71.

16. Ibid; see also Program for the Fifth Annual Conference of Texas Foundations and Trust Funds, Houston, Texas, April 15, 1953, Box MAI9-U21, Hogg Foundation Papers.

17. Program for the Seventh Annual Conference of Texas Foundations and Trust Funds, Dallas, Texas, April 19–20, 1955, Box MAI9-U21, Hogg Foundation Papers.

18. Program for the Eleventh Annual Conference of the Conference of Southwest Foundations, Santa Fe, New Mexico, April 1959, Box MAI9-U21, Hogg Foundation Papers.

19. Program for the Fifteenth Annual Conference of the Conference of Southwest Foundations, Dallas, Texas, April 1963, Box MAI9-U21, Hogg Foundation Papers.

20. Program for the Sixteenth Annual Conference of the Conference of Southwest Foundations, Albuquerque, New Mexico, April 1964; Program for the Eighteenth Annual Conference of the Conference of Southwest Foundations, Ardmore, Oklahoma, April 1966, Box MAI9-U21, Hogg Foundation Papers.

21. Program for the Twentieth Annual Conference of the Conference of Southwest Foundations, San Antonio, Texas, April 1968, Box MAI9-U21, Hogg Foundation Papers.

22. Program for the Twenty-Third Annual Conference of the Conference of Southwest Foundations, Kerrville, Texas, April 1971, Box MAI9-U21, Hogg Foundation Papers.

23. Program for the Twenty-Eighth Annual Conference of the Conference of Southwest Foundations, Nuevo Laredo, Tamaulipas, Mexico, April 1976; Program for the Thirtieth Annual Conference of the Conference of Southwest Foundations, El Paso, Texas, and Juarez, Mexico, April 1978, Box MAI9-U21, Hogg Foundation Papers.

24. Kelley, *The Foundations of Texas Philanthropy*, 70–71; Kirkland, *The Hogg Family and Houston*, 117; "The Conference of Southwest Foundations," Box MAI9-U21, Hogg Foundation Papers.

25. Kelley, *The Foundations of Texas Philanthropy*, 72.

26. Author interview with Wayne Holtzman, November 21, 2013.

27. Author interview with Lucille DiDomenico, March 31, 2014.

28. Ibid; Kelley, *The Foundations of Texas Philanthropy*, 73. The Conference of Southwest

Foundations relocated to Dallas in 1996–97, when Lucille DiDomenico assumed the role of executive director.

29. Author interview with Lucille DiDomenico, March 31, 2014.

30. Ibid.

31. Ira Iscoe, *Women View Their Working World: Based on a Study in Mental Health for the Texas Federation of Business and Professional Women* (Austin, TX: Hogg Foundation for Mental Health, 1963), Box MAI9-U34, Hogg Foundation Papers. This discussion also draws on author interview with Ira and Louise Iscoe, December 5, 2013.

32. Kelley, *The Foundations of Texas Philanthropy*, 73; author interview with Lucille DiDomenico, March 31, 2014.

33. This backlash is summarized in Kelley, *The Foundations of Texas Philanthropy*, 67–68 and 77–79.

34. "Probe Fails to Consider Good Works by Groups," *Fort Worth Star Telegram*, April 1, 1963.

35. The full nine-part series was reprinted as "Texas Foundations," undated pamphlet c. 1963, Box MAI9-U21, Hogg Foundation Papers.

36. Maud Keeling, *The Patman Committee, the Treasury Report, and Federal Grants: A Report of Interviews with Thirty Southwest Foundations* (Austin, TX: Conference of Southwest Foundations, fall 1967), Box MAI9-U21, Hogg Foundation Papers.

37. Kelley, *The Foundations of Texas Philanthropy*, 68.

38. Ibid., 78–79.

39. Curriculum vitae for Robert Lee Sutherland, 1959, Box MAI9-U23, Hogg Foundation Papers.

40. *Annual Report of the Hogg Foundation for Mental Health, 1961–62*, 11–12.

41. Wayne H. Holtzman, "Executive Director's Report: Sixty Years of Mental Health Philanthropy," *Annual Report of the Hogg Foundation for Mental Health, 1999–2000*.

42. Robert L. Sutherland and Wayne H. Holtzman, "The Unfolding of an Idea: The Hogg Foundation for Mental Health," *The Graduate Journal*, 1.2 (Fall 1958), 182–86. The article was reprinted and distributed as a pamphlet by the Foundation in 1964.

43. Ibid.

44. Ima Hogg to Judge Scott Gaines, November 17, 1949; Ima Hogg to John A. McCurdy, Texas Ex-Students Association, November 17, 1949; Ima Hogg to Robert L. Sutherland, November 17, 1949; Ima Hogg to Robert L. Sutherland, February 5, 1951; Ima Hogg to Robert L. Sutherland, September 24, 1951, Box MAI9-U1, Hogg Foundation Papers.

45. Ima Hogg to Robert L. Sutherland, April 5, 1950, Box MAI9-U1, Hogg Foundation Papers.

46. Ima Hogg to Dudley K. Woodward, July 5, 1952, Box MAI9-U1, Hogg Foundation Papers.

47. Meeting Minutes, University of Texas Board of Regents, July 11–12, 1952. Will C. Hogg Memorial Fund, Board of Regents Minutes (1939–59), University of Texas System Archives. The original figure also appeared in the Hogg family entry in the university's 1950 prospectus, "Developing a University Second to None," Box 3B122–3B123, Ima Hogg Papers.

48. Ima Hogg to Dudley K. Woodward, supra note 44.

49. Meeting Minutes, University of Texas Board of Regents, October 5, 1953. Will C. Hogg Memorial Fund, Board of Regents Minutes (1939–59), University of Texas System Archives.

50. Robert L. Sutherland to Ima Hogg, May 18, 1962. Will C. Hogg Memorial Fund, Accounting & Correspondence (History File), University of Texas System Archives. On

clinical research, see Logan Wilson to Robert L. Sutherland, June 2, 1954, Box MAI9-U28, Hogg Foundation Papers.

51. Unabridged Report of Meeting of Advisory Committees from the Texas Psychological Association and the Texas Neuropsychiatric Association to the Hogg Foundation for Mental Hygiene, December 12, 1953, Box MAI9-U23, Hogg Foundation Papers.

52. Robert L. Sutherland, Meeting Summaries, Texas Social Welfare Association Advisory Committee, January 27, 1951; Texas Neuropsychiatric Association Advisory Committee, January 23, 1950, and September 15, 1951; Texas Psychological Association Advisory Committee, April 6, 1950; April 28, 1951; September 29, 1951; and April 24, 1952; and Texas State Teachers College Liaison Committee, April 28, 1952, Box MAI9-U23, Hogg Foundation Papers.

53. "Memorandum: Research Policy Program of the Hogg Foundation, 1952," August 25, 1952; Sutherland, "Notes on Meeting with Dr. Paul White, Dr. Wayne Holtzman, and Dr. Beatrix Cobb," July 17, 1953, Box MAI9-U25, Hogg Foundation Papers; Ima Hogg to Robert L. Sutherland, November 5, 1952, Box MAI9-U1, Hogg Foundation Papers.

54. Unabridged Report of Meeting of Advisory Committees, supra note 50.

55. Robert L. Sutherland, "Notes on Meeting with Dr. Paul White, Dr. Wayne Holtzman, and Dr. Beatrix Cobb," July 17, 1953; "Memorandum: Based on Conference with Dr. Wilson, Concerning Policies in the Hogg Foundation Program," July 21, 1953; Sutherland, "Memorandum to Persons and Departments Involved in Mental Health Research," June 9, 1954, Box MAI9-U25, Hogg Foundation Papers.

56. Meeting Minutes, University of Texas Board of Regents, October 29, 1954. Will C. Hogg Memorial Fund Files, Board of Regents Minutes (1939–59), University of Texas System Archives. On Foundation budgets to that point, see *The Hogg Foundation Reports: Twelve Years of Mental Health Work in Texas* (Austin, TX: Hogg Foundation of Mental Health, January 1953).

57. Author interview with Wayne H. Holtzman, November 12, 2013.

58. Ibid.

59. Prominent examples of "culture and personality" studies include Margaret Mead, *Coming of Age in Samoa: A Psychological Study of Primitive Youth* (New York: William Morrow and Co., 1928); Ruth Benedict, *Patterns of Culture* (New York: Houghton Mifflin Harcourt, 1934); and Karen Horney, *The Neurotic Personality of Our Time* (New York: W.W. Norton & Co., 1937). Historical discussions of the culture and personality school include Nathan Hale Jr., *The Rise and Crisis of Psychoanalysis in the United States: Freud and the Americans, 1917–1985* (Cambridge, MA: Harvard University Press, 1995), and Philip Cushman, *Constructing the Self, Constructing America: A Cultural History of Psychotherapy* (Reading, MA: Addison-Wesley, 1995), 186–92.

60. Author interview with Wayne Holtzman, November 12, 2013.

61. "Memorandum Concerning Advisory Conference," April 19, 1955, Box MAI9/U23, Hogg Foundation Papers.

62. Ibid.

63. Ibid.

64. Memo, Robert Sutherland to Members of Advisory Committees, undated, c. spring 1955, Box MAI9/U23, Hogg Foundation Papers.

65. Sutherland, "Material Prepared for the Hogg Foundation Staff Meeting," July 11, 1955, Box MAI9/U23, Hogg Foundation Papers.

66. In 1958–59, research made up $114,426 of $247,167; subsequent figures are as fol-

lows: $154,697 of $345,000 (1960–61), $151,800 of $345,000 (1961–62), $128,973 of $345,000 (1963–64). *Annual Reports of the Hogg Foundation for Mental Health, 1958 to 1964.*

67. Sutherland, "Material Prepared for the Hogg Foundation Staff Meeting," supra note 64.

68. Sutherland and Holtzman, "The Unfolding of an Idea," 185.

69. Ibid., 186.

70. Harry Estill Moore, *Tornadoes Over Texas: A Study of Waco and San Angelo in Disaster* (Austin: University of Texas Press, 1958).

71. Ibid; see also Roy Sylvan Dunn, "Tornadoes," *Handbook of Texas Online* (Austin: Texas State Historical Association), http://www.tshaonline.org/handbook/online/articles/ydt01 (accessed July 20, 2014).

72. Joseph B. Perry Jr., "*Tornadoes Over Texas: A Study of Waco and San Angelo in Disaster* and Its Impact on the Study of Disaster," *International Journal of Mass Emergencies and Disasters*, 6.3 (November 1988): 253–81 (esp. 270). Perry was a former graduate student in sociology at the University of Texas who had served as one of Moore's research assistants.

73. Robert A. Stallings, "Weberian Political Sociology and Sociological Disaster Studies," *Sociological Forum*, 17.2 (June 2002): 281–305 (esp. 285).

74. Moore, *Tornadoes Over Texas*, chapter 7 (esp. 250–51).

75. Most recently, see James R. Elliott and Jeremy Pais, "When Nature Pushes Back: Environmental Impact and the Spatial Redistribution of Socially Vulnerable Populations," *Social Science Quarterly*, 91.5 (December 2010): 1187–1202, which notes that more recent studies of disasters have focused on how "socially disadvantaged residents" often suffer the most during disasters and disaster relief efforts.

76. Questions for Consultants' Consideration, Meeting Notes, National Advisory Committee Meeting, Hogg Foundation for Mental Health, May 25–26, 1959, Box MAI9-U132, Hogg Foundation Papers.

77. Wayne H. Holtzman, Joseph S. Thorpe, Jon D. Swartz, and E. Wayne Herron, *Inkblot Perception and Personality* (Austin, TX: University of Texas Press, 1961).

78. Daniel E. Sheer, ed., *Electrical Stimulation of the Brain: An Interdisciplinary Survey of Neurobehavioral Integrative Systems* (Austin: University of Texas Press, 1961).

79. Carl F. Hereford, *Changing Parental Attitudes Through Group Discussion* (Austin: University of Texas Press, 1963); Frances Merchant Carp, *A Future for the Aged: Victoria Plaza and Its Residents* (Austin: University of Texas Press, 1966); Arthur J. Rubel, *Across The Tracks: Mexican-Americans in a Texas City* (Austin: University of Texas Press, 1966).

80. Stephen J. Whitfield, *The Culture of the Cold War*, 2d ed. (Baltimore, MD: Johns Hopkins University Press, 1996); for an overview in Texas, see Don E. Carleton, *Red Scare: Right-Wing Hysteria, Fifties Fanaticism, and Their Legacy in Texas* (Austin: University of Texas Press, 2014).

81. Originally published in *Harper's Magazine* in 1964, the essay appears in Richard Hofstadter, *The Paranoid Style in American Politics and Other Essays* (New York: Vintage Books, 1967).

82. On Cvetic's mental health activism, see Daniel J. Leab, *I Was a Communist for the F.B.I.: The Unhappy Life and Times of Matt Cvetic* (University Park: Pennsylvania State University Press, 2000), 120–23. The quotes come from Matt Cvetic, "The Mental Health Goldbrick," *The American Mercury*, 88 (March 1959): 123–26.

83. Heather Hendershot, *What's Fair on the Air? Cold War Right-Wing Broadcasting and the Public Interest* (Chicago: University of Chicago Press, 2011), 65–101.

84. Ibid; see also Margaret L. Hartley, "Whose Mental Health? The Psychology of Suspicion," *Southwest Review* 46.4 (Fall 1961). Perhaps reflecting the fringe nature of these groups,

conservative Arizona Senator Barry Goldwater helped the Alaska Mental Health Act gain passage after it had been stalled by these criticisms.

85. Fred Schwarz, "Communism . . . A Disease!" brochure, 1959; "Mental Health: A Few Questions and Answers," Canadian Intelligence Service brochure, November 1959; Institute for Public Service brochure, February 1960; Newsletter, Texans for America Not Incorporated, A Committee for Political Action, March 15, 1961; Alan Duckworth, "Basic Subjects Termed Neglected," *Dallas Morning News*, March 28, 1961, Box MAI9-U23, Hogg Foundation Papers.

86. Proceedings of the Midcentury White House Conference on Children and Youth, December 3–7, 1950 (Raleigh, NC: Health Publications Institute, 1951), 266–68. On Erikson's talk, which marked one of his first public statements of his theory of identity crisis, see Lawrence J. Friedman, *Identity's Architect: A Biography of Erik H. Erikson* (Cambridge, MA: Harvard University Press, 1999), 220–29.

87. Bernice Milburn Moore and Wayne H. Holtzman, *Tomorrow's Parents: A Study of Youth and Their Families* (Austin: University of Texas Press, 1965), 3.

88. Ibid., 114. General conclusions are summarized on pages 8–9. For specific data on black teenagers, see pages 113–28; on social class and education, see pages 255–78. The book's theoretical framework melds 1950s ego psychology with late 1950s and early 1960s urban sociology. For example, while the book's body sections tend to focus extensively on individual "adjustment" to a presumed middle-class norm, the final chapter relies on "opportunity theory"—an approach that guided 1960s "community action" antidelinquency programs—to explain why certain families failed to socialize their children into "normal" middle-class society. On opportunity theory, see Richard A. Cloward and Lloyd E. Ohlin, *Delinquency and Opportunity: A Theory of Delinquent Gangs* (Chicago: University of Chicago Press, 1960). An earlier publication of some survey results focuses almost entirely on "adjustment" issues. Wayne H. Holtzman and Bernice Milburn Moore, "What Texas Knows About Youth," *National Parent-Teacher* (September 1958): 22–24.

89. Don E. Carleton, *Red Scare! Right-Wing Hysteria, Fifties Fanaticism, and Their Legacy in Texas* (Austin: University of Texas Press, 1985); see also William Henry Kellar, *Make Haste Slowly: Moderates, Conservatives, and School Desegregation in Houston* (College Station: Texas A&M University Press, 1999).

90. Unless otherwise noted, the following vignette comes from these reports written by Wayne Holtzman, Associate Director, Hogg Foundation: "The Nature and Purposes of the Houston Youth Study," June 12, 1959; and "Interim Report of Houston Youth Study," June 26, 1959, Box MAI9-U23, Hogg Foundation Papers.

91. Houston Youth Study test booklet, April 1959, Box MAI9-U23, Hogg Foundation Papers.

92. "The Nature and Purposes of the Houston Youth Study," June 12, 1959, Box MAI9-U23, Hogg Foundation Papers.

93. Houston Youth Study test booklet, April 1959, Box MAI9-U23, Hogg Foundation Papers.

94. Editorial, *Houston Chronicle*, June 10, 1959, Box MAI9-U23, Hogg Foundation Papers.

95. Houston Youth Study test booklet, April 1959, Box MAI9-U23, Hogg Foundation Papers.

96. On *Brown*'s legacy for psychology, race, and the South, see Glenn Adams, Monica Biernat, Nyla R. Branscombe, Christian S. Crandall, and Lawrence S. Wrightsman, eds., *Commemorating Brown: The Social Psychology of Racism and Discrimination* (Washington, DC: American Psychological Association, 2008); Daryl Michael Scott, *Contempt and Pity:*

Social Policy and the Image of the Damaged Black Psyche, 1880–1996 (Chapel Hill: University of North Carolina Press, 1997). On White, see Kellar, *Make Haste Slowly*, 109–12.

97. Untitled news clippings, *Houston Press*, June 4 and June 6, 1959, Box MAI9-U23, Hogg Foundation Papers.

98. "Interim Report of Houston Youth Study," June 26, 1959, Box MAI9-U23, Hogg Foundation Papers.

99. "Subversive Program Sneaked Into Houston Schools Is Thrown Out by Irate Parents," *The Southern Conservative* (undated newsletter, c. June 1959). News clipping, Box MAI9-U23, Hogg Foundation Papers.

100. Ima Hogg to Robert L. Sutherland, June 15, 1959, Box MAI9-U1, Hogg Foundation Papers.

101. Memo, Robert L. Sutherland to Wayne H. Holtzman, February 22, 1960, with handwritten reply from Holtzman written in margins, Box MAI9-U23, Hogg Foundation Papers.

102. Alan Duckworth, "Basic Subjects Termed Neglected," *Dallas Morning News*, March 28, 1961.

103. Newsletter, Texans for America Not Incorporated, A Committee for Political Action, March 15, 1961, Box MAI9-U23, Hogg Foundation Papers.

104. Memo, Robert L. Sutherland to Hogg Foundation staff, April 5, 1961, Box MAI9-U23, Hogg Foundation Papers.

105. Ibid.

106. "Interview with Miss Ima Hogg," November 21, 1961, Box MAI9/U25, Hogg Foundation Papers.

107. Ibid.

108. Copy of Meeting Minutes, University of Texas Board of Regents, March 8, 1962, Box MAI9/U25, Hogg Foundation Papers.

109. Ima Hogg to Harry Ransom, May 28, 1962, Box 4W254, Ima Hogg Papers.

110. The following discussion, with quotations, draws from Meeting Agenda and Meeting Transcript, Hogg Foundation National Advisory Council, June 26, 1961, Box MAI9-U132, Hogg Foundation Papers.

Chapter 5

1. Ann Salfield to Bert Kruger Smith, February 15, 1967, Box BKS 3A210/45, Hogg Foundation Papers.

2. Gerald N. Grob, *From Asylum to Community: Mental Health Policy in Modern America* (Princeton, NJ: Princeton University Press, 1991), 181–208.

3. Ibid.

4. Ibid., 210.

5. Erving Goffman, *Asylums: Essays on the Social Situation of Mental Patients and Other Inmates* (New York: Anchor Books, 1961); Howard S. Becker, *Outsiders: Studies in the Sociology of Deviance* (New York: The Free Press, 1963).

6. Grob, *From Asylum to Community*, 240–49.

7. Ibid., 267–70.

8. Ibid., 257.

9. Brochure, "Texas Research League Analyzes, No. 5: Significance of Constitutional Amendment Number Seven," October 1, 1956. Josephine Lamb Collection, 1954–66, Archives and Information Services Division, Texas State Library and Archives.

10. Hogg Foundation for Mental Health newsletter, spring 1958, Hogg Foundation Vertical Files.

11. C. Lincoln Willison, Texas Medical Association, to Robert L. Sutherland, September 13, 1957, Box MAI9-U29, Hogg Foundation Papers.

12. "Some Pertinent Comments Made on the Rehabilitation Study of the Hogg Foundation with Robert L. Sutherland, Glenn Rollins, Wayne Holtzman, Charles Laughton and Bernice Moore Participating," December 31, 1957, Box MAI9-U29, Hogg Foundation Papers.

13. "Notes from Conference Held March 1, 1958," Box MAI9-U29, Hogg Foundation Papers.

14. Ibid.

15. Ibid.; "Mental Health," *Odessa American*, March 1, 1959.

16. Ibid.

17. Fred R. Crawford, Glen W. Rollins, and Robert L. Sutherland, "Variations in the Evaluation of the Mentally Ill," *Journal of Health and Human Behavior*, 1 (Fall 1960): 211–19.

18. Fred R. Crawford, Glen W. Rollins, and Robert L. Sutherland, "Variations in the Evaluation of the Mentally Ill, Part II" *Journal of Health and Human Behavior*, 2 (Winter 1961): 267–75.

19. The following discussion draws from "Kaleidoscope," excerpts attached to Robert L. Sutherland to Wayne H. Holtzman, March 1, 1960, Box MAI9-U29, Hogg Foundation Papers.

20. Fred R. Crawford, Glen W. Rollins, and Robert L. Sutherland, "Variations Between Negroes and Whites in Concepts of Mental Illness and Its Treatment," *Annals of the New York Academy of Sciences*, 84 (December 1960): 918–37.

21. Glen W. Rollins, "Reports on the Mentally Ill (Big Spring)," 1959, Box MAI9-U29, Hogg Foundation Papers.

22. Ira Iscoe, "Editorial: The Final Report of the Joint Commission on Mental Health and Illness: Implications for Clinical Psychology," *Journal of Clinical Psychology* (May 1962): 110.

23. *The Texas Plan for Mental Health Services*, prepared by the Statewide Citizens Committee for Mental Health Planning, December 1, 1964, 11.

24. Meeting Notes, State Mental Health Planning Committee, Steering Committee, February 2, 1963, Box MAI9-U35, Hogg Foundation Papers.

25. *Annual Report of the Hogg Foundation for Mental Health, 1963–64*.

26. Meeting Notes, State Mental Health Planning Committee, Steering Committee, March 15, 1963, Box MAI9-U35, Hogg Foundation Papers.

27. Ibid.

28. "The Texas Plan for Comprehensive Mental Health Program Planning," May 1, 1963, Box MAI9-U36, Hogg Foundation Papers.

29. Meeting Notes, State Mental Health Planning Committee, Steering Committee, June 8, July 13, and August 16, 1963, Box MAI9-U35, Hogg Foundation Papers.

30. "The Future Is Now: Statewide and Community Planning for Mental Health Services," Office of Mental Health Planning, Texas State Department of Health, October 11, 1963, Box MAI9-U35, Hogg Foundation Papers.

31. Ibid.

32. Ibid.

33. Meeting Notes, State Mental Health Planning Committee, Steering Committee, October 26 1963, Box MAI9-U35, Hogg Foundation Papers.

34. Remarks of Governor John Connally, Texas Association for Mental Health, Dallas, Texas, October 18, 1963, Box MAI9-U35, Hogg Foundation Papers.

35. Ibid.

36. Memo, "Task Force Composition," Mental Health Planning, General Planning Committee, July 8, 1963, Box MAI9-U35, Hogg Foundation Papers.

37. Archie R. Foley, "Discussion on Mental Health Planning," October 15, 1963, Box MAI9-U35, Hogg Foundation Papers.

38. Ibid.

39. Questionnaire from Office of Mental Health Planning, January 27, 1964; Fred R. Crawford, "Comparison of Mental Health Research Grants—Texas and California," Special Memorandum, Office of Mental Health Planning Research Staff to Members of Research Task Force, March 31, 1964; "Fact Sheet on Social Work Manpower and Social Work Education, 1963–64," May 4, 1964; "1964 Salary Range Comparisons of Psychiatric Social Work Positions and Psychologist Positions (limited)," June 5, 1964, Box MAI9-U35, Hogg Foundation Papers.

40. Fred R. Crawford, Research Memorandum Number 3, Office of Mental Health Planning, to members of the General Planning Committee, March 31, 1964, Box MAI9-U35, Hogg Foundation Papers.

41. "Mental Health Treatment Resources in the 21 Major Population Centers," July 1964, Box MAI9-U35, Hogg Foundation Papers.

42. "Comments Regarding Administration and Coordination of the Texas Plan," Services to Troubled People Task Force, September 15, 1964, Box MAI9-U35, Hogg Foundation Papers.

43. *The Texas Plan for Mental Health Services.*

44. Memo, Robert L. Sutherland to Moody Bettis, undated, c. August 1964, Box MAI9-U35, Hogg Foundation Papers.

45. Memo, Moody Bettis to General Planning Committee, December 4, 1964, Box MAI9-U35, Hogg Foundation Papers.

46. "Mental Cases: City Walk-In Clinics Considered for Texas," *Austin Statesman*, October 16, 1963.

47. "Oswald Case Spurs Mental Health Push," *Austin Statesman*, December 10, 1963; also, "One of Last Official Acts: Kennedy's Mental Health Plan Lauded," *Fort Worth Star-Telegram*, December 9, 1963.

48. "Mental Health Planning in Texas," radio script, Texas State Department of Health, September 22, 1963, Box MAI9-U35, Hogg Foundation Papers; "Treatment: Survey Shows Mental Health Centers Needed in 21 Texas Cities," *Austin Statesman*, September 13, 1964.

49. Memo, Chairman to Mental Health Executive Committee, February 26, 1965, Box MAI9-U36, Hogg Foundation Papers.

50. "Mental Health Department Bill Becomes Law," *Houston Post*, April 6, 1965; and "Prevention of Disease is Stressed" and "Boost Forecast in Mental Care," *Austin American-Statesman*, April 15, 1965.

51. Dennis R. Jones and Sheila Allee, "Texas Department of Mental Health and Mental Retardation," *Handbook of Texas Online* (Austin: Texas State Historical Society), http://www.tshaonline.org/handbook/online/articles/mctvf (accessed October 23, 2013).

52. On the grants, see *Annual Report of the Hogg Foundation for Mental Health, 1964–65* and *1966–67*.

53. *Annual Report of the Hogg Foundation for Mental Health, 1964–65.*

54. Ibid.

55. Ima Hogg to Robert L. Sutherland, January 6, 1958, Box MAI9-U1, Hogg Foundation Papers.

56. *Annual Report of the Hogg Foundation for Mental Health, 1963–64.*

57. For a full accounting of Houston Action for Youth, see William S. Bush, "Representing the Juvenile Delinquent: Reform, Social Science, and Teenage Troubles in Postwar Texas," PhD. dissertation, University of Texas, 2004, chapter 3. For primary documents regarding Sutherland's role, see Box 3M390, Sutherland Papers.

58. Page Keeton to Norman Hackerman, April 20, 1966; Hackerman to Robert L. Sutherland, April 28, 1966; Sutherland to Louis Tomaino, Associate Director, Southwest Center, March 22, 1967; "HEW Grant Application for the Southwest Center Project, 1967–1968," Sutherland to Dr. Harold J. Belgum, February 22, 1971, Box 3M390, Sutherland Papers.

59. "Professor Bob Dawson, In His Own Words," excerpt from an oral history interview (2004). University of Texas School of Law website, http://www.utexas.edu/law/news/2005/dawson_interview.html (accessed June 30, 2005).

60. Robert L. Sutherland to Ima Hogg, October 5, 1970; Ira Iscoe to Hogg, February 26, 1971; Sutherland to Hogg, March 29, 1971; Wayne Holtzman to Hogg, July 14, 1972; Holtzman to Hogg, August 1, 1972; Sutherland to Hogg, October 30, 1973; Sutherland to Hogg, November 12, 1974, Box MAI9-U25, Hogg Foundation Papers.

61. Corrinne S. Tsanoff, "Working Together for Neighborhood Improvement," *Children* 11:5 (September–October 1964), 179–82 (esp.180); "Study of the Clayton Homes Neighborhood Development Program: A Total Neighborhood Approach," project proposal submitted by the Neighborhood Centers Association of Houston and Harris County to the National Institutes of Health, December 4, 1961, Box 3M390, Sutherland Papers.

62. "Study of the Clayton Homes Neighborhood Development Program," Box 3M390, Sutherland Papers.

63. "Creating a Neighborhood Climate for Better Mental Health," talk given to the Boston Settlement Council, July 1963; "Settlement Programs with Mental Health Implications for Urban Areas," talk given to the National Institutes of Mental Health, August 1963, Papers of Franklin Israel Harbach, Houston Metropolitan Research Center, Houston Public Library.

64. Ima Hogg to Robert L. Sutherland, January 6, 1959, Box MAI9-U23, Hogg Foundation Papers.

65. Harry Ransom to Robert L. Sutherland, January 28, 1958, Box MAI9-U23, Hogg Foundation Papers.

66. Robert L. Sutherland to J.R. Rees, December 4, 1963; Rees to Sutherland, November 25, 1963; Sutherland to David Hunter, Ford Foundation, December 2, 1963, Box MAI9-U14, Hogg Foundation Papers. Oswald's life history, including his psychiatric diagnosis while in a juvenile reformatory in New York, is described in chapter 7 of *Warren Commission, Report on the Assassination of President Kennedy* (New York: McGraw-Hill, 1964), 375–429. For a recent discussion, see Stephen A. Diamond, "Why Did Lee Harvey Oswald Kill John Fitzgerald Kennedy?" *Psychology Today,* November 21, 2013.

67. Pamphlet and press release, "Nightmare at Noon," September 7, 1966; and, Bert Kruger Smith, "Trio at a Tragedy," undated, c. fall 1966, Box 3A211, Hogg Foundation Papers.

68. On the Whitman incident, see Gary M. Lavergne, *The Sniper in the Tower. The Charles Whitman Murders* (Denton: University of North Texas Press, 1997); on Whitman's session with Heatly, see pages 70–73. For a shorter summary, see Alwyn Barr, "Whitman,

Charles Joseph," *Handbook of Texas Online,* http://www.tshaonline.org/handbook/online/articles/fwh42 (accessed January 25, 2014).

69. "Whitman Drawn to Famed Tower," *Houston Chronicle,* August 7, 1966.

70. Quote from Texas Governor's Committee and Consultants, *The Charles J. Whitman Catastrophe,* September 8, 1966, 9–10; for a summary of its findings, see Lavergne, *The Sniper in the Tower,* 254–71.

71. Robert L. Sutherland to Nicholas Hobbs, May 24, 1965; Meeting Notes, National Advisory Committee, Hogg Foundation for Mental Health, January 7–8, 1965, Box MAI9-U133, Hogg Foundation Papers.

72. Memo on Conference with Rabbi Levi Olan and His Committee, April 21, 1966, Box 3M380, Sutherland Papers.

73. Levi A. Olan to Robert L. Sutherland, May 20, 1966; Meeting Notes, Vice-Chancellor's Committee on Counseling Services, June 7, 1966, Box 3M380, Sutherland Papers.

74. Meeting Notes, Vice-Chancellor's Committee on Counseling Services, July 20, 1966, Box 3M380, Sutherland Papers.

75. Memo, Ira Iscoe to Robert L. Sutherland, July 22, 1966, Box 3M380, Sutherland Papers.

76. Author interview with Ira and Louise Iscoe, December 5, 2013.

77. Ibid.; Distinguished Service Award speech, American Psychological Association, Washington, D.C., 1976, Box MAI9-U18, Hogg Foundation Papers.

78. Memo, Ira Iscoe to Robert L. Sutherland, August 31, 1966, Box 3M380, Sutherland Papers.

79. Ira Iscoe report, "The Philosophy of Intake: Counseling Service, UCLA," undated, c. August 1966, Box 3M380, Sutherland Papers.

80. Report of the Vice-Chancellor's Committee on Counseling Services, September 26, 1966, Box 3M380, Sutherland Papers.

81. Memo, Robert L. Sutherland to Members of the Vice-Chancellor's Committee on Counseling Services, September 12, 1966; Meeting Notes, Vice-Chancellor's Committee on Counseling Services, September 13 and October 3, 1966, Box 3M380, Sutherland Papers.

82. Meeting Notes, Vice-Chancellor's Committee on Counseling Services, January 12, 1967; Memo, Harry Ransom to the Board of Regents, March 10, 1967, Box 3M380, Sutherland Papers.

83. Interim Report of the Counseling Committee, University of Texas YMCA and YWCA, March 1967; Meeting Notes, YM-YW Meeting, March 17, 1967, Box 3M380, Sutherland Papers.

84. Texas Governor's Committee and Consultants, *The Charles J. Whitman Catastrophe: Follow-Up Study on Recommendations,* September 8, 1967, Box 3K435, Iscoe (Ira) Papers, 1966–84, Dolph Briscoe Center for American History, University of Texas at Austin.

85. Memo, Ira Iscoe to Robert L. Sutherland, May 15, 1968, Box 3M380, Sutherland Papers.

86. Ira Iscoe quote, from author interview with Ira and Louise Iscoe, December 5, 2013.

87. The following discussion draws on Ira Iscoe, Director, Counseling and Psychological Services Center, University of Texas at Austin, "The Development and Evaluation of Innovative Mental Health Services within a University Counseling Center Framework," November 1968, Box BKS 2.35-W41, Hogg Foundation Papers; and "Volunteer's Handbook, The Listening Ear," 1970, Hogg Foundation for Mental Health Vertical Files.

88. Memo, Robert L. Sutherland to National Advisory Council, January 6, 1967, Box MAI9-U18, Hogg Foundation Papers.

Chapter 6

1. Harry Ransom to Robert L. Sutherland, June 20, 1970, Box MAI9-U14, Hogg Foundation Papers.

2. Homer P. Rainey, "A Personal Reminiscence," in *The Hogg Foundation for Mental Health: The First Three Decades* (Austin: University of Texas, 1970), 3–5.

3. "A Letter from Miss Ima," in *The Hogg Foundation for Mental Health*, 1–2.

4. Ernest E. Neal to Robert L. Sutherland, February 11, 1971, Box MAI9-U14, Hogg Foundation Papers.

5. Loyd Rowland to Bernice Moore, June 13, 1970, Box MAI9-U14, Hogg Foundation Papers.

6. There is a voluminous literature on the antipoverty community action projects of the 1960s, much of which debates whether or not they were successful. See Alice O'Connor, *Poverty Knowledge: Social Science, Social Policy, and the Poor in the Twentieth-Century U.S. History* (Princeton, NJ: Princeton University Press, 2001), 124–138; Annelise Orleck and Lisa Gayle Hazirjian, eds., *The War on Poverty: A New Grassroots History, 1964–1980* (Athens: University of Georgia Press, 2011); Irwin Unger, *The Best of Intentions: The Triumphs and Failures of the Great Society Under Kennedy, Johnson, and Nixon* (New York: Doubleday, 1996), 54–69; Thomas F. Jackson, "The State, the Movement, and the Urban Poor: The War on Poverty and Political Mobilization in the 1960s," in Michael B. Katz, ed., *The "Underclass" Debate: Views From History* (Princeton, NJ: Princeton University Press, 1993), 403–39; and Allen J. Matusow, *The Unraveling of America: A History of Liberalism in the 1960s* (New York: Harper & Row, 1984), 108–19.

7. Recent studies include William S. Clayson, *Freedom is Not Enough: The War on Poverty and the Civil Rights Movement in Texas* (Austin: University of Texas Press, 2010); and, Brian D. Behnken, *Fighting Their Own Battles: Mexican Americans, African Americans, and the Struggle for Civil Rights in Texas* (Chapel Hill: University of North Carolina Press, 2011), esp. 154–95.

8. On the Chicano movement in Texas, see David Montejano, *Quixote's Soldiers: A Local History of the Chicano Movement, 1966–1981* (Austin: University of Texas Press, 2010); for a more general history, see Carlos Muñoz, *Youth, Identity, and Power: The Chicano Movement*, rev. ed. (New York: Verso Books, 2007 [1990]).

9. Author interview with Wayne Holtzman, November 21, 2013; curriculum vitae for Wayne Holtzman; Robert L. Sutherland to Maude Keeling, April 20, 1970, Box MAI9-U14, Hogg Foundation Papers.

10. *Annual Report of the Hogg Foundation for Mental Health, 1964–65, 1965–66.*

11. *Annual Report of the Hogg Foundation for Mental Health, 1970–71.*

12. William Madsen, *Society and Health in the Lower Rio Grande Valley* (Austin, TX: Hogg Foundation for Mental Health, 1961), preface.

13. Ibid., 30–35.

14. Carl M. Rosenquist and Edwin I. Megargee, *Delinquency in Three Cultures* (Austin: University of Texas Press, 1969), preface and 127–29.

15. Ibid., 136–42.

16. Ibid., 463. On the "culture of poverty," see Oscar Lewis, *Five Families: Mexican Case Studies in the Culture of Poverty* (New York: New American Library, 1959); and O'Connor, *Poverty Knowledge*, 99–124.

17. Wayne H. Holtzman, Rogelio Díaz-Guerrero, and Jon D. Swartz, *Personality Develop-*

ment in Two Cultures: A Cross-Cultural Longitudinal Study of School Children in Mexico and the United States (Austin: University of Texas Press, 1975).

18. Review by Eugene Jacobson, *Annals of the American Academy of Political and Social Science*, 389 (May 1970): 174–75; review by John Casparis, *American Sociological Review*, 35.5 (October 1970): 975–77; review by A.F. Gailly, *International Journal of Psychology*, 12.1 (March 1977): 66–68; review by David J. Ellingson, *Journal of Personality Assessment*, 41.3 (June 1977): 324–26.

19. Robert L. Sutherland to David V. Edwards, March 27, 1969, Box MAI9-U17, Hogg Foundation Papers.

20. *Annual Report of the Hogg Foundation for Mental Health, 1970–71.*

21. Memo, Robert L. Sutherland to National Advisory Council members, November 22, 1965, Box MAI9-U133, Hogg Foundation Papers.

22. Meeting Minutes, National Advisory Council, Hogg Foundation, December 9–10, 1968; Bert Kruger Smith, "Eastside Community Involvement Project," December 1968, Box MAI9-U133, Hogg Foundation Papers.

23. Meeting Minutes, National Advisory Council, Hogg Foundation, June 9–10, 1969, Box MAI9-U134; and, Jack Otis to Stan Brown, June 1, 1969, Box MAI9-U14, Hogg Foundation Papers.

24. Ibid.

25. "Ethnic Group Dilemmas and the Hogg Foundation Program," A Tentative Outline for Discussion, National Advisory Council, Hogg Foundation, January 21–22, 1971, Box MAI9-U134, Hogg Foundation Papers.

26. Ibid.

27. Ibid.

28. Ibid.

29. "National Advisory Council Considers Prison Reform, Minority Group Programs," *The Hogg Foundation News*, 5.1 (Spring 1971): 1.

30. Meeting Minutes, National Advisory Council, Hogg Foundation, January 21–22, 1971, Box MAI9-U134, Hogg Foundation Papers.

31. Ibid.

32. *Hogg Foundation News*, 14.1 (Fall 1979): 4.

33. Author interview with Reymundo Rodríguez, February 26, 2014.

34. Author interview with Ralph Culler, January 30, 2014.

35. Author interview with Reymundo Rodríguez, February 26, 2014.

36. Much of this section relies on Sally Jones Andrade, *Chicano Mental Health: The Case of Cristal* (Austin, TX: Hogg Foundation for Mental Health, 1978).

37. Biographical Sketch, Erasmo, and Sally J. Andrade Papers, Benson Latin American Collection, University of Texas Libraries, University of Texas at Austin.

38. See Behnken, *Fighting Their Own Battles*, 176–81; Montejano, *Quixote's Soldiers*, xx.

39. Jose Angel Gutiérrez, *A Gringo Manual on How to Handle Mexicans*, 2d ed. (Houston, TX: Arte Público Press, 2001 [1974]), 73–76; this passage also appears in Andrade, *Chicano Mental Health*, 4.

40. Ibid, 76.

41. Andrade, *Chicano Mental Health*, 14.

42. Ibid., 15.

43. Author interview with Wayne Holtzman, November 12, 2013.

44. Andrade, *Chicano Mental Health*, 15–17.

45. Author interview with Reymundo Rodríguez, February 26, 2014.

46. Andrade, *Chicano Mental Health,* 34–40; Meeting Minutes, National Advisory Council, Hogg Foundation for Mental Health, December 16–18, 1973, Box MAI9-U135, Hogg Foundation Papers.

47. Author interview with Reymundo Rodríguez, February 26, 2014.

48. Andrade, *Chicano Mental Health,* 46.

49. Ibid., 62.

50. Ibid., 76.

51. Author interview with Reymundo Rodríguez, February 26, 2014.

52. Andrade, *Chicano Mental Health,* 93–102.

53. "Summary of 1973–1974 Grant Funds Through December 13, 1973," Meeting Minutes, National Advisory Council, Hogg Foundation for Mental Health, December 16–18, 1973, Box MAI9-U135, Hogg Foundation Papers.

54. Richard G. Frank and Sherry A. Glied, *Better But Not Well: Mental Health Policy in the United States Since 1950* (Baltimore, MD: Johns Hopkins University Press, 2006), 48–60.

55. Gerald N. Grob, "Public Policy and Mental Illnesses: Jimmy Carter's Presidential Commission on Mental Health," *The Milbank Quarterly,* 83.3 (September 2005): 425–56.

56. Ibid.

57. Ibid.

58. These activities are summarized in *Annual Reports of the Hogg Foundation for Mental Health, 1981 to 1986.*

59. Texas Legislative Council, *Summary of Enactments, 69th Legislature, Regular and First Called Sessions,* Information Report No. 85–4 (September 1985), 188–90.

60. Ibid.; Frank and Glied, *Better But Not Well,* 60–69.

61. *Annual Report of the Hogg Foundation for Mental Health, 1980–81.*

62. *Annual Report of the Hogg Foundation for Mental Health, 1983–84.*

63. *Annual Report of the Hogg Foundation for Mental Health, 1982–83,* for example, suggests that Ima Hogg opposed the Foundation becoming a "research foundation." In this budget, research amounts to about 17 percent of expenditures, in contrast to 44 percent in 1961–62.

64. *Annual Report of the Hogg Foundation for Mental Health, 1981–82,* Introduction.

65. *Annual Report of the Hogg Foundation for Mental Health, 1999–2000,* describes the Evaluation Research Program as "one of the first of its kind" and a model for program evaluation.

66. Author interview with Ralph Culler, January 30, 2014; the Casa de Esperanza appears in the *Annual Reports of the Hogg Foundation for Mental Health, 1983–1991.*

67. Author interview with Ralph Culler, January 30, 2014.

68. Among the Commission reports are the following: *Financing Community Care for the Chronically Mentally Ill in Texas* (1990); *Texas Children* (1990); *Technology, Training, Collaboration* (1990); *Reaching Out to Youth* (1990); *Choices Limited: Child Care for Children with Special Needs* (1989); *Community Mental Health in Texas: Four Case Studies* (1990); *Texans with Severe Mental Illness* (1990); *Texas Teens: The Status of Adolescents* (1990); and *Children, Choices, and Change* (1990). Of the several School of the Future publications, the clearest is the report on longer term outcomes: Louise K. Iscoe and Scott S. Keir. *Revisiting the School of the Future: The Evolution of a School-Based Services Project* (Austin, TX: Hogg Foundation for Mental Health, 1997).

69. Author interview with Wayne Holtzman, November 21, 2013.

70. *Annual Report of the Hogg Foundation for Mental Health, 2000–1.*

Epilogue

1. "Hogg Foundation for Mental Health Announces New Directions," Press Release, University of Texas at Austin, February 24, 2004.

2. Author interview with King L. Davis, April 24, 2014. For more on Joseph Bevilacqua, who served as commissioner of mental health in three states, see his biographical entry under "National Association of Social Workers Pioneers," http://www.naswfoundation.org/pioneers/default.asp (accessed April 30, 2014).

3. Ibid.

4. American Psychiatric Association Presidential Task Force on Evidence-Based Practice, "Evidence-Based Practice in Psychology," *American Psychologist*, 61.4 (May–June 2006): 271–85; Institute for the Advancement of Social Work Research, *Partnerships to Integrate Evidence-Based Mental Health Practices into Social Work Education and Research: A Report From April 12, 2007, Symposium Sponsored by the National Institute for Mental Health* (Washington, DC: IASWR, October 2007).

5. Author interview with King L. Davis, April 24, 2014.

6. "Language Matters in Mental Health," Hogg Foundation for Mental Health website, http://www.hogg.utexas.edu/initiatives/language_matters.html (accessed February 19, 2015).

Bibliography

Archival Collections

Bert Kruger Smith Papers, 1955–2004. Dolph Briscoe Center for American History, University of Texas at Austin.

Chairmen Lanning, Logan, Ashley, and Baker files. Texas State Board of Control Board members files. Archives and Information Services Division, Texas State Library and Archives Commission.

Franklin Israel Harbach Papers. Houston Metropolitan Research Center, Houston Public Library.

Hogg Foundation for Mental Health Records, 1872–. Dolph Briscoe Center for American History, University of Texas at Austin.

Ima Hogg Papers, 1824–1977. Dolph Briscoe Center for American History, University of Texas at Austin.

Ira Iscoe Papers, 1966–84. Dolph Briscoe Center for American History, University of Texas at Austin.

Josephine Lamb Collection, 1954–66. Archives and Information Services Division, Texas State Library and Archives Commission.

Robert Lee Sutherland Papers, 1937–73. Dolph Briscoe Center for American History, University of Texas at Austin.

Texas Board for Texas State Hospitals and Special Schools records. Archives and Information Services Division, Texas State Library and Archives Commission.

University of Texas President's Office Papers, 1907–68. Dolph Briscoe Center for American History, University of Texas at Austin.

Will C. Hogg Fund, Accounting & Correspondence (History File). University of Texas System.

Will C. Hogg Memorial Fund Files, Board of Regents Minutes (1939–59). University of Texas System.

Reference Sources

Handbook of Texas

Legislative Reference Library of Texas (http://www.lrl.state.tx.us/index.cfm).

Vertical Files. Dolph Briscoe Center for American History, University of Texas at Austin.

Oral Interviews

Ralph Culler, January 30, 2014.
King Davis, April 24, 2014.
Lucille DiDomenico, March 31, 2014.
Adrian Fowler, April 3, 2015.
Wayne Holtzman, November 12, 2013.
Ira and Louise Iscoe, December 5, 2013.
Robert Léon, April 17, 2014.
Reymundo Rodríguez, February 26, 2014.

Newspapers and Periodicals

Abilene Reporter-News
Amarillo News-Globe
Austin American-Statesman
Baytown Sun Daily
Beaumont Journal
Bellville Times Weekly
Big Spring Herald Daily
Bryan Daily Eagle
CNN
Corsicana Sun
Cuero Daily Record
Daily Texan
Dallas Morning News
DeLeon Free Press
El Campo News
El Paso Times
Fort Worth Star-Telegram
Fort Worth Weekly
Galveston News
Harlingen Valley Morning Star
Hillsboro Evening Mirror
Houston Chronicle
Houston Post
Houston Press
Junction Eagle
Kilgore News Herald
Longview News-Journal
Los Angeles Times
Lubbock Avalanche
Marshall News Messenger
New York Daily News
North Texas American
Odessa American
Palestine Herald-Press
Paris Daily News
Rockdale Reporter
San Angelo Standard-Times
San Antonio Express News
San Jacinto Times
Texas Tribune
Think Progress
Tyler Morning Telegraph
Waco Tribune Herald
Wichita Daily Times
Yahoo News

Published Historical Sources

Andrade, Sally Jones. *Chicano Mental Health: The Case of Cristal.* Austin, TX: Hogg Foundation for Mental Health, 1978.

"An Idea Worth Fulfilling: History of the School of Social Work, 1950–1983." Austin: University of Texas School of Social Work, 2010.

Annual Reports of the Hogg Foundation for Mental Health, 1940–.

Becker, Howard S. *Outsiders: Studies in the Sociology of Deviance.* New York: The Free Press, 1963.

Beers, Clifford W. *A Mind That Found Itself: An Autobiography.* Garden City, NY: Doubleday, 1948. (Originally published 1908)

Carp, Frances Merchant. *A Future for the Aged: Victoria Plaza and Its Residents.* Austin: University of Texas Press, 1966.

Cloward, Richard A., and Lloyd E. Ohlin. *Delinquency and Opportunity: A Theory of Delinquent Gangs.* Chicago: University of Chicago Press, 1960.

Crawford, Fred R., Glen W. Rollins, and Robert L. Sutherland. "Variations Between Negroes and Whites in Concepts of Mental Illness and Its Treatment." *Annals of the New York Academy of Sciences,* 84 (December 1960): 918–37.

Cvetic, Matt. "The Mental Health Goldbrick." *The American Mercury,* 88 (March 1959).

Deutsch, Albert. *The Shame of the States.* New York: Harcourt, Brace, and Co., 1948.

Goffman, Erving. *Asylums: Essays on the Social Situations of Mental Patients and Other Inmates.* Garden City, NY: Anchor Books, 1961.

Gutiérrez, Jose Angel. *A Gringo Manual on How to Handle Mexicans,* 2d ed. Houston, TX: Arte Público Press, 2001. (Originally published 1974)

Hamilton, Samuel W. "Life in Our Mental Hospitals: Its Meaning for the Individual." *Mental Hygiene,* 27.1 (January 1943): 3–9.

Hamilton, Samuel W. *Survey of State Mental Institutions of Texas.* Austin: Texas State Board of Control, 1943.

Hartley, Margaret L. "Whose Mental Health? The Psychology of Suspicion." *Southwest Review,* 46.4 (Fall 1961).

Hereford, Carl F. *Changing Parental Attitudes Through Group Discussion.* Austin: University of Texas Press, 1961.

Holtzman, Wayne H., Rogelio Diaz-Guerrero, and Jon D. Swartz. *Personality Development in Two Cultures: A Cross-Cultural Longitudinal Study of School Children in Mexico and the United States.* Austin: University of Texas Press, 1975.

Holtzman, Wayne H., Joseph S. Thorpe, Jon D. Swartz, and E. Wayne Herron. *Inkblot Perception and Personality.* Austin: University of Texas Press, 1961.

Iscoe, Ira. "Editorial: The Final Report of the Joint Commission on Mental Health and Illness: Implications for Clinical Psychology." *Journal of Clinical Psychology* (May 1962): 110.

Iscoe, Ira. *Women View Their Working World: Based on a Study in Mental Health for the Texas Federation of Business and Professional Women.* Austin, TX: Hogg Foundation for Mental Health, 1963.

Iscoe, Louise K., and Scott S. Keir. *Revisiting the School of the Future: The Evolution of a School-Based Services Project.* Austin, TX: Hogg Foundation for Mental Health, 1997.

Lewis, Oscar. *Five Families: Mexican Case Studies in the Culture of Poverty.* New York: New American Library, 1959.

Lumpkin, Joseph Howard. "Group Counseling and the Learning of Teacher Roles." PhD dissertation, University of Texas at Austin, 1954.

Madsen, William. *Society and Health in the Lower Rio Grande Valley.* Austin, TX: Hogg Foundation for Mental Health, 1961.

Moore, Bernice Milburn, and Wayne H. Holtzman. *Tomorrow's Parents: A Study of Youth and Their Families.* Austin: University of Texas Press, 1965.

Moore, Harry Estill. *Tornadoes Over Texas: A Study of Waco and San Angelo in Disaster.* Austin: University of Texas Press, 1958.

Rockwood, Edith, and Augusta J. Street. "Social Protective Work of Public Agencies, With Special Emphasis on the Policewoman." Washington, DC: League of Women Voters, August 1932.

Rosenquist, Carl M., and Edwin I. Megargee. *Delinquency in Three Cultures.* Austin: University of Texas Press, 1969.

Rubel, Arthur J. *Across The Tracks: Mexican-Americans in a Texas City.* Austin: University of Texas Press, 1966.

Ruud, Millard H. *Interpretation of the Mental Health Code,* 1st ed. Austin: University of Texas, 1957.

Sheer, Daniel E., ed. *Electrical Stimulation of the Brain: An Interdisciplinary Survey of Neurobehavioral Integrative Systems.* Austin: University of Texas Press, 1961.

Smith, Bert Kruger, dir. *In a Strange Land.* Austin, TX: Hogg Foundation for Mental Health, 1956.

Stone, Susan. *Recommendations for Updating the Texas Mental Health Code: A Response to Decades of Dramatic Change in Texas' Mental Health System.* Austin: Texas Appleseed, September 2012.

Sutherland, Robert L. "Relation Between Eschatology and Jesus' Ethics." MA thesis, Oberlin College, August 1927.

Sutherland, Robert L. "An Analysis of Negro Churches in Chicago." PhD dissertation, University of Chicago, 1930.

Sutherland, Robert L. *Color, Class, and Personality.* Washington, DC: American Council on Education, 1942.

Sutherland, Robert L. "Society's Responsibility for Protecting the Mental Health of Children." *Texas State Journal of Medicine,* 37 (February 1942): 658–61.

Sutherland, Robert L. *Essentials of a Community Mental Health Program: Tentative Guideposts for Community Planning.* Austin: Hogg Foundation for Mental Hygiene, November 1945.

Sutherland, Robert L., and Wayne Holtzman, "The Unfolding of an Idea." *Graduate Journal,* 1.2 (Fall 1958).

The Hogg Foundation for Mental Health: The First Three Decades. Austin: University of Texas Press, 1970.

The Hogg Foundation Reports: A Summary of Three Years Work, A Forecast of Next Steps. Austin: University of Texas Press, February 1944.

The Hogg Foundation Reports: Twelve Years of Mental Health Work in Texas. Austin: University of Texas Press, 1953.

The Texas Plan for Mental Health Services. Prepared by the Statewide Citizens Committee for Mental Health Planning. December 1, 1964.

Zurcher, Louis A. Jr. *Poverty Warriors: The Human Experience of Planned Social Intervention.* Austin: University of Texas Press, 1970.

Secondary Sources

Adams, Glenn, Monica Biernat, Nyla R. Branscombe, Christian S. Crandall, and Lawrence S. Wrightsman, eds. *Commemorating Brown: The Social Psychology of Racism and Discrimination.* Washington, DC: American Psychological Association, 2008.

Anderson, Greta. *More Than Petticoats: Remarkable Texas Women.* Guilford, CT: Globe Pequot Press, 2002.

Bailey, Beth L. *From Front Porch to Back Seat: Courtship in Twentieth Century America.* Baltimore, MD: Johns Hopkins University Press, 1989.

Behnken, Brian D. *Fighting Their Own Battles: Mexican Americans, African Americans, and the Struggle for Civil Rights in Texas.* Chapel Hill: University of North Carolina Press, 2011.

Bernhard, Virginia, ed. *The Hoggs of Texas: Letters and Memoirs from an Extraordinary Family, 1887–1906*. Denton: Texas State Historical Association, 2013.

Blanton, Carlos Kevin. "The Campus and the Capitol: John B. Connally and the Struggle Over Texas Higher Education Policy, 1950–1970." *Southwestern Historical Quarterly*, 108.4 (April 2005): 468–97.

Bills, E.R. *The 1910 Slocum Massacre: An Act of Genocide in East Texas*. Charleston, SC: The History Press, 2014.

Brightman, Mikel Jean Fisher. "An Historical Survey of the State of Texas' Efforts to Aid the Mentally Ill and the Mentally Retarded." MA thesis, University of Texas, 1971.

Bush, William S. "Representing the Juvenile Delinquent: Reform, Social Science, and Teenage Troubles in Postwar Texas." PhD dissertation, University of Texas, 2004.

Bush, William S. *Who Gets a Childhood? Race and Juvenile Justice in Twentieth Century Texas*. Athens: University of Georgia Press, 2010.

Cahn, Susan K. *Sexual Reckonings: Southern Girls in a Troubling Age*. Cambridge, MA: Harvard University Press, 2007.

Campbell, Randolph B. *Gone to Texas: A History of the Lone Star State*. New York: Oxford University Press, 2003.

Carleton, Don E. *Red Scare: Right-Wing Hysteria, Fifties Fanaticism, and Their Legacy in Texas*. Austin: University of Texas Press, 2014. (Originally published 1985)

Clayson, William S. *Freedom Is Not Enough: The War on Poverty and the Civil Rights Movement in Texas*. Austin: University of Texas Press, 2010.

Cotner, Robert. *James Stephen Hogg, A Biography*. Austin: University of Texas Press, 1959.

Cushman, Philip. *Constructing the Self, Constructing America: A Cultural History of Psychotherapy*. Reading, MA: Addison-Wesley, 1995.

Dugger, Ronnie. *Our Invaded Universities: Form, Reform, and New Starts*. New York: Norton, 1974.

Evans, Richard I., ed. *The Making of Social Psychology: Discussions with Creative Contributors*. New York: Gardner Press, 1980.

Frank, Richard G., and Sherry A. Glied. *Better But Not Well: Mental Health Policy in the United States Since 1950*. Baltimore, MD: Johns Hopkins University Press, 2006.

Friedman, Lawrence J. *Identity's Architect: A Biography of Erik H. Erikson*. Cambridge, MA: Harvard University Press, 1999.

Grob, Gerald N. *Mental Illness and American Society, 1875–1940*. Princeton, NJ: Princeton University Press, 1983.

Grob, Gerald N. *From Asylum to Community: Mental Health Policy in Modern America*. Princeton, NJ: Princeton University Press, 1991.

Grob, Gerald N. *The Mad Among Us: A History of the Care of America's Mentally Ill*. New York: The Free Press, 1994.

Grob, Gerald N. "Public Policy and Mental Illnesses: Jimmy Carter's Presidential Commission on Mental Health." *The Milbank Quarterly*, 83:3 (September 2005): 425–56.

Grob, Gerald N., ed. *Public Policy and Mental Illness: Four Investigations, 1915–1939*. New York: Arno Press, 1980.

Hale, Nathan Jr. *The Rise and Crisis of Psychoanalysis in the United States: Freud and the Americans, 1917–1985*. Cambridge, MA: Harvard University Press, 1995.

Hendershot, Heather. *What's Fair on the Air? Cold War Right-Wing Broadcasting and the Public Interest*. Chicago: University of Chicago Press, 2011.

Herman, Ellen. *The Romance of American Psychology: Political Culture in an Age of Experts*. Berkeley: University of California Press, 1995.

Hofstadter, Richard. *The Paranoid Style in American Politics and Other Essays.* New York: Vintage Books, 1967.

Horn, Margo. *Before It's Too Late: The Child Guidance Movement in the United States, 1922–1945.* Philadelphia: Temple University Press, 1989.

Iscoe, Louise. *Ima Hogg: First Lady of Texas.* Austin: Hogg Foundation for Mental Health, 1976.

Jones, Kathleen W. *Taming the Troublesome Child: American Families, Child Guidance, and the Limits of Psychiatric Authority.* Cambridge, MA: Harvard University Press, 1999.

Kellar, William Henry. *Make Haste Slowly: Moderates, Conservatives, and School Desegregation in Houston.* College Station: Texas A&M University Press, 1999.

Kelley, Mary L. *The Foundations of Texas Philanthropy.* College Station: Texas A&M University Press, 2004.

Kirkland, Kate Sayen. *The Hogg Family and Houston: Philanthropy and the Civic Ideal.* Austin: University of Texas Press, 2009.

Lavergne, Gary M. *The Sniper in the Tower: The Charles Whitman Murders.* Denton: University of North Texas Press, 1997.

Leab, Daniel J. *I Was a Communist for the F.B.I.: The Unhappy Life and Times of Matt Cvetic.* University Park: Pennsylvania State University Press, 2000.

Lomax, John Avery. *Will Hogg, Texan.* Austin: Hogg Foundation for Mental Health, 1956. (Originally published 1940)

May, Elaine Tyler. *Homeward Bound: American Families in the Cold War Era.* New York: Basic Books, 1988.

Miller, Char L., and Heywood T. Sanders, eds. *Urban Texas: Politics and Development.* College Station: Texas A&M University Press, 1990.

Montejano, David. *Quixote's Soldiers: A Local History of the Chicano Movement, 1966–1981.* Austin: University of Texas Press, 2010.

Muñoz, Carlos. *Youth, Identity, and Power: The Chicano Movement*, rev. ed. New York: Verso Books, 2007. (Originally published 1990)

Neeley, Gwendolyn Cone. *Miss Ima and the Hogg Family.* Dallas: Hendrick-Long, 1992.

Nelson, Geoffrey, Bret Kloos, and José Ornelas, eds. *Community Psychology and Community Mental Health: Towards Transformative Change.* New York: Oxford University Press, 2014.

O'Connor, Alice. *Poverty Knowledge: Social Science, Social Policy, and the Poor in the Twentieth-Century U.S. History.* Princeton, NJ: Princeton University Press, 2001.

Orleck, Annelise, and Lisa Gayle Hazirjian, eds. *The War on Poverty: A New Grassroots History, 1964–1980.* Athens: University of Georgia Press, 2011.

Palladino, Grace. *Teenagers: An American History.* New York: Basic Books, 1998.

Perry, Joseph B. Jr. "*Tornadoes Over Texas: A Study of Waco and San Angelo in Disaster* and Its Impact on the Study of Disaster." *International Journal of Mass Emergencies and Disasters*, 6.3 (November 1988): 253–81.

Pickren, Wade E., and Stanley F. Schneider, eds. *Psychology and the National Institute for Mental Health: A Historical Analysis of Science, Practice, and Policy.* Washington, DC: American Psychological Association, 2005.

Reston, James Jr. *The Lone Star: The Life of John Connally.* New York: HarperCollins, 1989.

Richardson, Theresa R. *The Century of the Child: The Mental Hygiene Movement and Social Policy in the United States and Canada.* Albany: State University of New York Press, 1989.

Rossinow, Douglas. *The Politics of Authenticity: Liberalism, Christianity, and the New Left in America.* New York: Columbia University Press, 1998.

Rothman, David J. *Conscience and Convenience: The Asylum and Its Alternatives in Progressive America*, 2d ed. New York: Aldine de Gruyter, 2002. (Originally published 1980)

Rothman, David J. *The Discovery of the Asylum: Social Order and Disorder in the New Republic*, rev. ed. New York: Aldine Transaction, 2002. (Originally published 1971)

Schrum, Kelly. *Some Wore Bobby Sox: The Emergence of Teenage Girls' Culture, 1920–1945.* New York: Palgrave Macmillan, 2004.

Scott, Daryl Michael. *Contempt and Pity: Social Policy and the Image of the Damaged Black Psyche, 1880–1996.* Chapel Hill: University of North Carolina Press, 1997.

Sitton, Sarah C. *Life at the Texas State Lunatic Asylum, 1857–1997.* College Station: Texas A&M University Press, 1999.

Storey, John W., and Mary L. Kelley eds. *Twentieth Century Texas: A Social and Cultural History.* Denton: University of North Texas Press, 2008.

The Hogg Foundation for Mental Health: The First Three Decades. Austin: University of Texas, 1970.

Tuttle, William M. Jr. *Daddy's Gone to War: The Second World War in the Lives of America's Children.* New York: Oxford University Press, 1993.

Whitfield, Stephen J. *The Culture of the Cold War*, 2d ed. Baltimore, MD: Johns Hopkins University Press, 1996.

Index